Critical Thinking and Writing for Nursing Students

Third Edition

Critical Thinking and Writing for Nursing Students

Bob Price
Anne Harrington

Series Editor: Mooi Standing

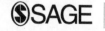

Los Angeles | London | New Delhi
Singapore | Washington DC

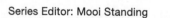

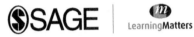

Learning Matters
An imprint of SAGE Publications Ltd
1 Oliver's Yard
55 City Road
London EC1Y 1SP

SAGE Publications Inc.
2455 Teller Road
Thousand Oaks, California 91320

SAGE Publications India Pvt Ltd
B 1/I 1 Mohan Cooperative Industrial Area
Mathura Road
New Delhi 110 044

SAGE Publications Asia-Pacific Pte Ltd
3 Church Street
#10-04 Samsung Hub
Singapore 049483

© Bob Price and Anne Harrington, 2010, 2013, 2016

First edition published 2010
Second edition 2013
Third edition 2016

Editor: Alex Clabburn
Development editor: Richenda Milton-Daws
Production controller: Chris Marke
Project management: Swales & Willis Ltd, Exeter, Devon
Marketing manager: Tamara Navaratnam
Cover design: Wendy Scott
Typeset by: C&M Digitals (P) Ltd, Chennai, India
Printed and bound by CPI Group (UK) Ltd, Croydon, CR0 4YY

Library of Congress Control Number: 2015951586

British Library Cataloguing in Publication data

A catalogue record for this book is available from the British Library

ISBN 978-1-4739-2507-6
ISBN 978-1-4739-2508-3 (pbk)

At SAGE we take sustainability seriously. Most of our products are printed in the UK using FSC papers and boards. When we print overseas we ensure sustainable papers are used as measured by the PREPS grading system. We undertake an annual audit to monitor our sustainability.

Contents

TRANSFORMING NURSING PRACTICE

TNP

Transforming Nursing Practice is a series tailor-made for pre-registration student nurses. Each book in the series is:

○ Affordable
○ Mapped to the NMC Standards and Essential Skills Clusters
○ Full of active learning features
○ Focused on applying theory to practice

Each book addresses a core topic and they have been carefully developed to be simple to use, quick to read and written in clear language.

"

An invaluable series of books that explicitly relates to the NMC standards. Each book cover a different topic that students need to explore in order to develop into a qualified nurse... I would recommend this series to all Pre-Registration nursing students whatever their field or year of study

Linda Robson
Senior Lecturer, Edge Hill University

The set of books is an excellent resource for students. The series is small, easily portable and valuable. I use the whole set on a regular basis.

Fiona Davies
Senior Nurse Lecturer, University of Derby

I recommend the SAGE/Learning Matters series to all my students as they are relevant and concise. Please keep up the good work.

Thomas Beary
Senior Lecturer in Mental Health Nursing, University of Hertfordshire

"

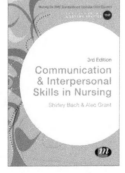

3rd Edition
Communication & Interpersonal Skills in Nursing
Shirley Bach & Alec Grant

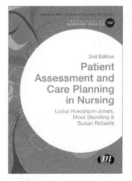

2nd Edition
Patient Assessment and Care Planning in Nursing
Lioba Howatson-Jones, Mooi Standing & Susan Roberts

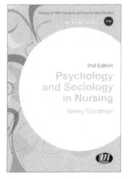

2nd Edition
Psychology and Sociology in Nursing
Benny Goodman

Foreword

The Transforming Nursing Practice series includes several titles which focus on personal and professional learning skills needed by nurses in order to deliver safe and effective care. Critical thinking and writing for nursing students addresses both of these areas by guiding readers in how to process information and then articulate what they have learned. Readers' personal development is facilitated in acquiring, understanding and demonstrating critical thinking, reflecting and scholarly writing skills. This goes hand-in-hand with professional development as readers are given useful tips on how to make use of the learning situations that they experience, and how to apply critical thinking in formal academic assessments. Readers are encouraged to engage with lots of interesting activities which combine and progressively stretch their personal and professional learning skills regarding critical thinking. The book utilises the experience of four nursing students during their nursing programme as a device to illustrate different perspectives and attributes of others learning to develop critical thinking skills. This offers a reference point for readers to gauge their own development in this respect. After reading this book nursing students and others will be well versed in the different components of critical thinking, how to demonstrate their use in classroom and clinical settings, and the importance of applying these skills to enhance patient care.

In the third edition of this well received book, the authors have incorporated changes which take account of new developments, feedback and their continued commitment in making a complex topic understandable and helpful to readers. For example, they show how critical thinking skills enable nurses to fulfil their professional duties as specified in *The Code: Professional standards of practice and behaviour for nurses and midwives* (NMC, 2015). In doing so they demonstrate that critical thinking/reflection is essential to relate the theory of delivering person centred, safe and effective nursing interventions to clinical practice. The authors provide a new framework to describe different levels of critical thinking in relation to different aspects of reflection. This is very helpful for nursing students to understand what is expected of them at different stages of their programme, and how they might achieve this. In updating *Critical Thinking and Writing for Nursing Students*, the authors have ensured that it remains an invaluable resource for nursing students, mentors and lecturers to refer to.

Dr Mooi Standing
Series Editor

Acknowledgements

We would like to gratefully acknowledge the contributions of Stewart, Fatima, Raymet and Gina, who very generously agreed to explore critical thinking and reflection with us through their own work. Thanks go too to Gavin McNally and Ali Saher, students of City University, Community Health Sciences Department, and Sally Thorpe, Academic Adviser, School of Nursing and Midwifery at City University, who kindly read a number of the chapters.

Finally, all authors owe a debt of gratitude to families who patiently wait while books are written. Irrespective of what the book is about, the wait is the same and the patience central to success. We are surrounded by supportive people. Thank you all.

About the authors

Bob Price is a healthcare education and training consultant. Formerly, he was Director, Postgraduate Awards in Advancing Healthcare Practice at the Open University. A passionate educator, Bob has assisted students at every level from pre-registration programmes of study up to and including Doctor of Philosophy. Bob's doctoral thesis was on the negotiation of learning and strategies used by students and tutors to develop scholarly and professional forms of expression.

Anne Harrington (formerly from City University) is senior lecturer in Ethics, Public Health, Mentor in Practice, Leadership and Management and Study Skills at Brighton University. Anne has been teaching for nearly 25 years, and is passionate about supporting and enhancing students' learning experience. Her PhD in Education focused on the students' experience of academic support in higher education and reported that many of them who had their prior academic education overseas found it difficult to develop critical and analytical thinking when writing their essays.

Guide to the companion website accompanying this book

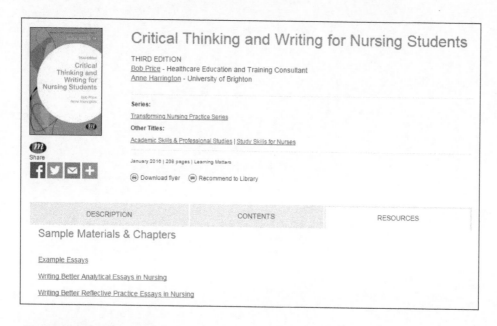

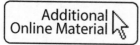

With critical thinking and writing, sometimes one of the best ways to improve your understanding is to look at some examples of how others have approached this. To help, the authors have supplied some sample essays – both reflective and analytical – that are available for you to download and read from the companion website.

Also available is detailed guidance and examples showing how to demonstrate higher levels of critical thinking and reflection in your work and practice.

To access the material visit www.sagepub.co.uk/price_harrington and click on the tab that says 'Resources'. From there you can access the essays completely free of charge.

Introduction

The ability to think critically, to reflect upon experience and then to write about such matters in a clear fashion is central to your success on a programme of nursing studies and, subsequently, the maintenance of professional standards in line with *The Code* for nurses and midwives (Nursing and Midwifery Council, 2015). This book is designed to assist you with this process – the making sense of things that you read, hear, observe and experience, its translation into learning and representation within academic forms of writing set by the university. While other texts exist that describe reasoning and reflection, this one locks these skills into the process of learning and writing. However skilled you are as a critical thinker or as a reflector on practice, such abilities avail you little if you are then unable to express your learning to others. Importantly, the book will help you to write analytically at the appropriate level within your course and to express yourself in ways that convey your compassion and care for patients. While academic levels may be expressed in different ways in different countries, what remains constant is the need to demonstrate a progression of your learning, which meets the requirements set within coursework assignments and module examinations. This book addresses the needs of pre-registration, undergraduate learners. If you study nursing at a postgraduate level, the principles of reasoning discussed within these pages will still apply, but the course requirements set for you will be more exacting. It is often the case there that your critical reasoning and reflection will have to operate with less information to hand. It is not that you necessarily use different reasoning processes, but rather that you must use sound reasoning and reflection under more exacting conditions. Postgraduate learners work with greater levels of ambiguity.

Nursing presents us with a flood of information – gleaned from lectures, demonstrations, seminars and workshops, programmes of reading electronic forum discussions and what you discover during clinical placements. All of this has to be processed, and turned into that which you can use as a nurse. Processing this information in the right way takes time and benefits from wise counsel. You will naturally wish to liaise closely with your tutors as part of this work. As you think about what you have learned, and as you prepare essays and reflective journals, and revise for assessments, we believe that this textbook, ever present and available for consultation, will prove valuable.

Who is this book for?

We have written this book for student nurses completing their undergraduate pre-registration course of studies. We also believe that nurses taking subsequent short specialist courses of study, where they must once again prepare academic papers and complete assessments, will also find it useful. Postgraduate learners, those completing a postgraduate diploma or master's degree might find it useful to dip into this book, refreshing their memory on principles of reasoning, but this is not a book written primarily for master's degree or doctoral students. While we regularly refer to the Nursing and Midwifery Council's *Standards for Preregistration Nursing Education* (Nursing and Midwifery Council, 2010), the book will, we believe, also serve well in other countries. Sound critical thinking and writing are of concern everywhere.

Because the book starts from basics, it is designed to reassure and support those who may not have studied for some while. We begin with the assumption that critical thinking, reflecting and writing are three of the craft skills of nursing. Safe, well-organised and high-quality nursing care depends on these skills. Our approach is based on our experience of designing and delivering open and flexible learning study materials, which might be worked through by a nurse planning for a course as well as by those who are already enrolled. The book draws upon our experience of assessing coursework at different levels of undergraduate learning and provides guidance on how to demonstrate more analytical and insightful thinking. While coursework assessments may vary and you must read the questions with care, what represents more analytical and more deeply reflective thinking and writing can be learned and is taught within these pages for use by you and your personal tutor. Because academic levels are expressed a little differently within different countries we have purposefully not entered into a discussion of those levels. It is our argument that assessors set assignment requirements with regard to national academic level standards and then it is the job of this book to help students to address the assignment tasks set. Broadly speaking, you should assume that the highest levels of critical thinking and reflection set out within this textbook equate to what you should expect to demonstrate by the end of your undergraduate nursing course. You will work up towards these. Tutors do not expect you to achieve the most sophisticated reasoning from the very start of your undergraduate course.

Much of what is best in nursing is defined by the way in which we deliver care as much as by what is provided. The way we listen, explore anxieties and needs or suggest solutions demonstrates care and compassion. Within a busy healthcare service, where financial and work pressures exist, it has never been more important for nurses to seem compassionate (Department of Health and NHS Commissioning Board, 2012). The revised code of conduct of the Nursing and Midwifery Council (2015) lays special emphasis upon compassionate care under registration requirements relating to 'prioritising people'. For this reason, reading this textbook will start you on a journey where you discover how best to use your experience in the service of others. This is a process that draws heavily upon making sense of practice, exploring what you believe is best within nursing care and planning future development that helps you express your thinking more effectively.

Critical thinking and reflecting

One of the earliest discoveries made by nurses during their courses of study is how often the word 'critical' appears in their work. In the clinical context, the word carries connotations of risk and the need for urgent intervention: a patient is critically ill, the next stage of treatment is critical (e.g. Odell, 2015). It can sometimes suggest that deterioration has set in or that we have not acted as proactively as we might. Used in this sense, the nurse quickly realises the need for precision and judgement, the requirement to do the right thing, in the right way and at the right time. In the academic context, 'critical' takes on several different meanings (Morrall and Goodman, 2013).

You are asked to 'critically discuss', to 'critically evaluate', to 'critically explore' a subject, and it slowly becomes apparent that to be critical involves different things depending on the teaching or assessment involved. For example, to be critical in this context might mean to discriminate between what is right and wrong, defensible and indefensible. However, it might also involve making judgements about what is influential. If you are preparing a reflective piece of course-work, then 'critical' often involves being introspective, examining afresh your beliefs, values and motives. Nurses need to be self-aware practitioners and to anticipate how their approach might impact on the feelings of patients and relatives. Unfortunately, not all nursing course assessments spell out the sense in which the term critical is being used, so it is sometimes necessary to check with your tutor what the assessment requirements are.

In this textbook, we use the term 'critical thinking' in a precise way. It describes the process by which we develop powers of analysis and investigation, and enhance our ability to discriminate what is relevant and to discern what might prove most helpful.

Critical thinking involves judgement and nurses are frequently assessed with regard to their ability to judge and demonstrate skills and make appropriate decisions (Pitt et al., 2015). A competent nurse is one who selects the relevant information to plan a course of action and then judges what is best to do in a given circumstance. The nurse has to be competent in managing risk. As well as this, the nurse needs to carry on learning and to grow professionally through experience (Clarke et al., 2010).

We are best placed to improve care where we have the capacity to reason what is not yet under-stood and what will enable us to be more imaginative, sensitive, respectful or efficient and effective in what we do.

While 'critical' is sometimes encountered in a more destructive form within practice (e.g., where practitioners belittle others' shortfalls), this is not the sense in which we will use it here. Indeed, we suggest that the individual who criticises without consideration of what is learned through the experience is not demonstrating either scholarship or professionalism.

It is likely that you have already engaged in reflection as part of previous studies and while grow-ing up. For example, at school you perhaps judged which subjects to take to examination, based on your past comfort with them in class. However, in nursing, reflection has a very important and specific role. It is strongly associated with the development of empathy; that is, the understanding and respect for the circumstances of others. Nurses need to be emotionally intelligent, to antici-pate how illness, treatment and care might seem to patients and how different courses of action might seem to professional colleagues. Rankin (2013) reminds us that such emotional intelli-gence is critical to nurses who work in teams to care for the public. Because nurses are asked to use their experience and their insights as part of nursing care, reflection takes on a special mean-ing. While at least some of your teaching in college starts with concepts or theories that describe the world of health care, much of what you learn through practice starts from episodes of care that are much more ambiguous. We have to make sense of what is going on and decide how best to proceed when at least some information is currently unavailable to us. In an important paper on the design of future healthcare services, Carr et al. (2011) emphasise the need to combine such reflection and evidence. Evidence alone will not secure the healthcare improvements that nurses and others strive for. The process of reflection then is central to nurses' learning and must be combined with theory in order to suggest how best to work next. It can tell us a great deal about our goals and values, beliefs and attitudes as well as what experience offers. Not surprisingly, then, both critical thinking and reflection are centre stage within this textbook. Critical thinking engages our reasoning as we ponder theories, arguments and debates, while reflection does the same as we contemplate experience.

How this book is set out

This text is set out in three parts. You will certainly benefit from reading it cover to cover, but it will also serve you when you wish to 'dip into' particular chapters later. Part 1 of the book consists of three chapters that introduce you in an accessible way to the key concepts that feature in this book: critical thinking, reflecting and scholarly writing. Securing a basic idea about what these concepts are all about will help you make a great deal more sense of what is asked of you within the nursing syllabus. Within Part 1 we introduce you to different levels of critical thinking and reflection, something that you will need to understand in order to address the learning outcomes of modules as you progress through a course.

Part 2 of the textbook concerns the use of reasoning and reflection within different contexts. We help you to understand what is involved in getting the most from lectures, demonstrations, seminars, workshops and clinical placements, and while using electronic media in your learning. There has been an exponential growth in the use of electronic media to teach nursing, and this is often collaborative in nature. Debates, discussions, seminars and student presentations all feature within electronic media, so guidance on thinking and reflecting here is important.

As explained in Chapter 5, watching others demonstrate a technique or skill could seem quite passive learning, but in fact you will need in turn to show what you can do and we help you to prepare for that event. A seminar is a different proposition, one that assumes that you have done some preliminary work and will then discuss that during the session. Reasoning and reflecting in practice involves a different approach again; you need to accommodate the public nature of this learning environment, to enquire with due respect for the work that is under way there. Studying the chapters in Part 2 of this book will help you to become a more effective gatherer and processor of nursing information. Other sources of helpful guidance on the application of reasoning and reflection are provided by Ellis (2013) on evidence-based practice, Sharples (2011) on practice-based learning and Standing (2014) on clinical judgement and decision making.

If Part 2 is about the process of learning, then Part 3 is about the process of expressing what you have learned. This part opens with a chapter that represents an important development in critical thinking – the use of questions to interrogate different sorts of evidence. During your nursing career, you will have access to a wide range of evidence of varying quality, so it is vital that you can reason to best effect here. We assist you with the matter of writing different sorts of essays (analytical and reflective) and with building a portfolio that helps you to demonstrate progress and plan future learning (Reed (2015) provides a helpful supplementary resource on portfolio development for nurses). While there are many forms that assessment can take in nursing courses, the principles of analytical and reflective writing remain seminal. Students frequently ask how their writing can demonstrate deeper reflection and more critical thinking. They are exercised by the need to demonstrate critical analysis rather than simply analysis. They want help to better understand what is meant by critical reflection rather than simply reflection. Accordingly, in this section we spend some time illustrating how you can demonstrate different levels of critical thinking, those that may be required in different stages of your course.

Learning features

Throughout the book, you will find activities that will help you to make sense of, and learn about, the material being presented by the authors.

Some activities ask you to reflect on aspects of practice, or your experience of it, or the people or situations you encounter. *Reflection* is an essential skill in nursing, and one that helps you to understand the world around you and often to identify how things might be improved. Other activities will help you develop key skills, such as your ability to *think critically* about a topic in order to challenge received wisdom, or your ability to *research a topic and find appropriate information and evidence*, and to be able to *make decisions* using that evidence in situations that are often difficult and time-pressured.

All the activities require you to take a break from reading the text, think through the issues presented and carry out some independent study, possibly using the internet. Remember, academic study will always require independent work; attending lectures will never be enough to be successful on your programme, and these activities will help to deepen your knowledge and understanding of the issues under scrutiny and give you practice at working on your own. You might want to think about completing these activities as part of your portfolio. After completing the activity, write it up in your portfolio in a section devoted to that particular skill, then look back over time to see how far you are developing.

Because we know that case study illustrations of scholarly writing can prove very helpful indeed, we have positioned two examples of essays (one analytical and one reflective) on the publisher's website (**www.sagepub.co.uk/price_harrington**). Each of these is free to download and for you to use as you think further about essay writing. Remember, though, that these are illustrations of writing, and you should ensure that you do not copy these and present them as your own work to the university, something that constitutes plagiarism. Universities use software that readily identifies work copied from the internet or past students' work and penalties for academic misconduct may be severe. The website also illustrates some paragraphs of writing at different levels of analysis and reflection. Students and tutors tell us how important this is. If you are to write in a more analytical way, a less descriptive manner, it is important to see examples of what is more analytical, what is more reflective. While it is natural to feel anxious, perhaps even apprehensive about your studies, working with this book and its case studies should significantly improve your chances of not only doing well on your course, but enjoying study as well.

NMC Standards for Pre-registration Nursing Education and Essential Skills Clusters

For those readers who are studying nursing courses within the UK, the NMC has established *Standards for Pre-registration Nursing Education*, which are standards of competence to be met by applicants to different parts of the register, and which it considers necessary for safe and effective practice. In addition to the competencies, the NMC has set out specific skills that nursing students must be able to perform at various points of an education programme. These are known as Essential Skills Clusters (ESCs). Critical thinking, reflection and writing have widespread relevance across all nursing competencies and ESCs. Therefore, we have, at the start of each chapter, identified those to which we think our material relates very closely, and which assist the reader to achieve the requirements for registration as a nurse.

This book includes the latest standards for 2010 onwards, taken from *Standards for Pre-registration Nursing Education* (NMC, 2010).

Preparing for the NMC (2015) code of professional practice standards

While this book assumes that in most instances you are not yet a registered nurse, it is important to think ahead to how your learning about reasoning and reflecting here might serve you well as you maintain the professional standards expected by the public and protected through the work of the Nursing and Midwifery Council (2015). In 2015, the Council published its revised code of practice standards for UK nurses and midwives and these lay special emphasis on the sort of reasoning that we teach you about in this textbook. *The Code* describes four areas of professional responsibility:

- prioritise people;
- practise effectively;
- preserve safety;
- promote professionalism and trust.

Prioritise people

Nurses are required to attend quickly, considerately, respectfully and compassionately to other people, the service users within health care and their colleagues in practice. Nurses must be able to analyse others' likely needs and concerns and to respect their confidentiality and individuality whilst doing so. It is important for nurses to listen to the experience of patients and what they have to relate about their expectations and experience of care. Within a complex and busy healthcare service, the needs of the patient and their individuality and dignity must not be neglected.

If you are to prioritise people successfully, it is vital that you learn to think critically about their situation and needs. A patient may not know all of their concerns, needs and risks immediately, so you will have to be adept at identifying patterns of behaviour, clinical presentations and requirements that they might soon have. Learning about how best to ask questions and to evaluate the information that you secure from them is a vital part of planning individualised care with patients. Chapter 1 in this textbook teaches you about critical thinking and Chapter 6 helps you build confidence in thinking in a more critical way when you learn in the practice setting. Clinical areas are rich learning environments so learning to think strategically here is important. Chapter 2 introduces you to reflection as a process. Much of what you learn about delivering care in an individualised way comes from learning directly with and from patients. Learning to reflect well is then a vital part of delivering care that makes patients and relatives feel that they matter. What worried the patient most? How will that help shape the explanations and the reassurance that I give?

Practise effectively

It is not enough that nurses are respectful and considerate towards patients; they must be effective as well. Healthcare resources, be they medicines, materials or the nurse's time, are scarce resources and must be used to best effect. To work effectively the NMC (2015) *Code* requires that nurses make the best possible use of evidence, that they communicate clearly, that they work cooperatively and that they share their skills and expertise with others. Clear and accurate records of care are important and nurses must stand ready to be accountable when they delegate decisions or tasks to others.

Critical thinking (Chapter 1) is important in efficient and effective practice. What will work best and why? What is the best order in which to do things? Why might it be better to act in one way than another? Chapter 8 helps you to better understand evidence, much of which may come from research, but case study experience or audit may be important sources of information too. When you practise, you will need to introduce evidence in a clear, understandable and sensitive way to patients. You will need to anticipate how it could seem to them. Although evidence may recommend a course of action, this may not seem the best or most desirable course of action to the patient, so reflection (Chapter 2) is important here as well. A nurse might need to 'sell' the benefits of a recommended course of action to a patient.

Preserve safety

Nurses have the potential to cause considerable harm as well as to do great good. With this in mind, *The Code* requires that nurses work within the limits of their competence and the protocols and policies established within healthcare organisations. They must be prepared to raise concerns where patients seem at risk and to intervene in emergencies where they have the requisite competence to do so. Nurses must be prepared to acknowledge mistakes or errors and to act quickly and collaboratively to mitigate these where possible.

Judging exactly what we know, and how confident this might make you feel, is important. What you read about in Chapter 1 (Critical thinking), Chapter 2 (Reflection) and what you learn about making a case in Chapter 3 (Scholarly writing) will prompt you to examine again what supports arguments, a course of action. Safety often relies upon judging when not to act, when it is better to consult or refer, and this in turn relies upon a willingness to examine why something seems a good idea. Critical thinking, reflection and case making are then important in making better and safer decisions.

Promote professionalism and trust

The NMC *Code* (2015) reminds nurses of their professional responsibility to uphold the reputation of the profession and their own status as a nurse. To this end they must act without favour and not accept loans or gifts which might otherwise influence their professional judgement or the reputation of the profession. They must respond promptly and considerately to complaints and they must exercise leadership as part of work promoting the wellbeing of patients and excellence in care standards. Registered nurses are expected to carry on learning, refining and improving their professional skills and mastering new knowledge or approaches to care that reflect what evidence has taught.

Being ready to examine complaints honestly, to confront suspect practice relies upon our judgement ability. What is excellent, what is suspect, what could lead to harm or difficulty for the patient? We will need to think objectively and critically (Chapter 1), to reflect on events, even though they cause us to revisit our own values and beliefs (Chapter 2). We will need to amass experience and to refer back to it in ways that enable us to draw good conclusions. Chapter 11 in this book introduces you to the benefits of building and maintaining a professional portfolio.

Part 1
Understanding thinking, reflecting and writing

Chapter 1
Critical thinking

NMC Standards for Pre-registration Nursing Education

This chapter addresses the following competencies.

Domain 1: Professional values

8. All nurses must practise independently, recognising the limits of their competence and knowledge. They must reflect on these limits and seek advice from, or refer to, other professionals where necessary.
9. All nurses must appreciate the value of evidence in practice, be able to understand and appraise research, apply relevant theory and research findings to their work, and identify areas for further investigation.

Domain 3: Nursing practice and decision making

Decision making must be shared with service users, carers and families and informed by critical analysis of a full range of possible interventions.

1. All nurses must use up-to-date knowledge and evidence to assess, plan, deliver and evaluate care, communicate findings, influence change and promote health and best practice. They must make person-centred, evidence-based judgements and decisions, in partnership with others involved in the care process, to ensure high quality care. They must be able to recognise when the complexity of clinical decisions requires specialist knowledge and expertise, and consult or refer accordingly.

Domain 4: Leadership, management and team working

4. All nurses must be self-aware and recognise how their own values, principles and assumptions may affect their practice. They must maintain their own personal and professional development, learning from experience, through supervision, feedback, reflection and evaluation.

Chapter aims

After reading this chapter, you will be able to:

- define critical thinking in your own practical terms using illustrations as necessary;
- with reference to different components of critical thinking, discuss why this skill is important in nursing;

(Continued)

(Continued)

- summarise different aptitudes associated with critical thinking;
- indicate your level of confidence associated with each of the aptitudes of critical thinking, noting those that you hope to develop further in the future;
- describe what constitutes more sophisticated forms of critical thinking.

Introduction

Decision making, leadership and ethical practice are all founded upon an ability to think critically. We use critical thought to select resources, to deploy knowledge and to evaluate evidence. We have all been involved in reasoning throughout our lives, but it is highly likely that a lot of that has been conducted without a great deal of scrutiny. Many of the past decisions that we have made have been managed in a tacit way; that is, without great analysis. To be successful nurses, though, we need to practise the skill of critical thinking in a more conscious way (Lovatt, 2014; Standing, 2014).

Not only do we need to discover what we have learned, we need to understand how we have learned it. In this way we equip ourselves with the means to go on learning, even when our formal education is complete. In this chapter, we first explore why critical thinking is important in nursing, before unpicking what critical thinking typically consists of. The chapter ends with some suggestions on how you can enhance your critical thinking.

To help you explore further, we now introduce you to four student nurses. We will be returning to Stewart, Fatima, Raymet and Gina periodically throughout the book, but the discussions in this chapter focus on some of their early course learning.

Activity 1.1   *Reflection*

Think about the extent to which you have consciously thought about some judgements in your life so far. Have some of the decisions been dealt with tacitly (Kothari et al., 2012) without careful scrutiny? Here are some examples that you could consider.

- Choosing nursing as a career.
- Revising for examinations.
- Starting a new relationship.
- Evaluating healthcare news events, those relating to the reported quality of care, for example.

While information overload may preclude conscious scrutiny of everything, has tacit reasoning served you well? Is there sometimes a case for more conscious and shared reasoning?

Defining critical thinking

What do we mean by critical thinking? As Lovatt (2014) notes, a definition is difficult to pin down and each represents something of a compromise. However, it seems important to share with you our opening premises. For us, critical thinking is:

A process, where different information is gathered, sifted, synthesised and evaluated, in order to under-stand a subject or issue. Critical thinking engages our intellect (the ability to discriminate, challenge and argue), but it might engage our emotions too. To think critically we need to take account of values, beliefs and attitudes that shape our perceptions. Critical thinking, then, is that which enables the nurse to function as a knowledgeable doer – someone who selects, combines, judges and uses information in order to proceed in a professional manner. Critical thinking is vital if we are to act strategically and to convey our care and compassion for others.

Why critical thinking is important

Four student nurses meet up over coffee to discuss some of the challenges of completing a nursing studies course. While their studies are interesting, they all acknowledge that learning can be difficult because of the critical thinking required.

Activity 1.2   *Reflection*

Look now at the accounts in the box below of critical thinking challenges reported by these students.

- Have you encountered similar concerns?
- Why do you think that making connections between teaching and practice (Stewart), managing uncertainty (Fatima), dealing with large volumes of information (Raymet) and knowing how, as well as what, to do (Gina) tells us about the importance of critical thinking in nursing?

Case study: Four accounts of critical thinking challenges

Stewart: 'I've realised not only that there is important theory to grasp, but that it isn't always simple to apply, to use it in practice. For example, pharmacology teaches you about anti-inflammatory drugs but there are lots of caveats about when you use those.'

Fatima: 'For me it's the uncertainty. I long for a right answer, something that I know is sure and correct, and a lot of what we're learning about – for instance ethics – isn't so clear cut.'

continued ... •

Raymet: *'I agree! But have you noticed just how much information there is? It's like they fill up your kit bag with everything you could ever want and then leave you to decide when to pull it out. The sheer volume is worrying.'*

Gina: *'I wouldn't disagree with any of those points. But have you noticed how important it is to understand processes as well as purposes? You quickly learn what you should do, but how to do it is something more complex. It's that which I find myself admiring nurses for.'*

You may already be empathising with these four, each of whom captures something about critical thinking in nursing. Nursing practice relies heavily on the skills of the nurse, and central among these is the ability to reason. Skills are made up of a series of component parts, and it is the way in which these are combined and used that determines how skilful the practice seems (Gobet, 2005; Gobet and Chassey, 2008; see Figure 1.1). Nurses develop templates in their own minds to determine how best to work, but practice constantly demands that we adjust these ideas, combining and recombining the different skill components in ways to suit prevailing conditions.

In the case study above, Stewart refers to the first of these components. While his first concerns are about the application of theory, this only becomes important because, without clear guidance on this, Stewart is unsure how best to proceed. If we are going to deliver good nursing care we have to know how to combine and apply information. We have to be able to declare certain things (as true, sound, proven, relevant) if we are to develop the confidence to proceed.

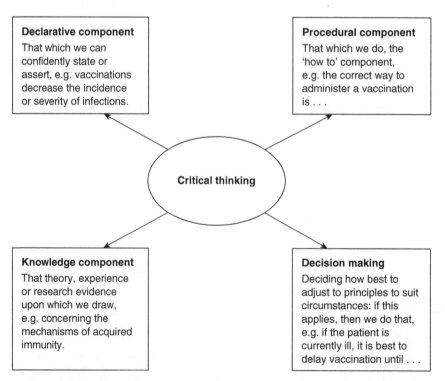

Figure 1.1: Components of nursing skill

Critical thinking in this context therefore involves the piecing together of bits of information from several different sources, in ways that help us to determine what is happening.

A very simple example makes the point. When Stewart cares for a patient receiving drugs to reduce inflammation, he would need to know something about the action of the chosen medication (theory), its effect on the physiology of the body (research evidence) and how this relates to patient need, in order to make sense of what to do next. Inflammation is one of the body's defence mechanisms, so suppressing inflammation is only a good idea when it is clear that the illness is understood, and any interactions with other drugs are taken into account. He could only declare what was normal, expected or problematic if he was able to combine and evaluate information in this way.

Fatima refers to a second important component of critical thinking, *decision making*. There is often no 'one size fits all' solution. Fatima is keenly aware that the nurse has to deal with uncertainty, sometimes waiting to gather more information before making a decision. Living with such uncertainty, especially in clinical practice, is what can seem stressful for nurses. They have to learn to read developing situations and to weigh the merits of different courses of action. The process of reasoning, therefore, is important to nursing because it provides a discipline for deciding how best to proceed in practice.

What Raymet is discussing concerns *knowledge*. Professional practice is underpinned by a raft of knowledge and this comes from many sources: research, experience, theory and work in related fields (e.g., counselling or medicine). We can only reason effectively if we have amassed a sufficient quantity of high-quality knowledge (Ellis, 2013a).

Reasoning, then, involves several things: accepting some sorts of knowledge as important, but standing ready to challenge others. As well as choosing what knowledge to use in practice, the nurse needs to know when to discard knowledge and search for something more robust. So, while Stewart is concerned with what information fits a particular situation (application), Raymet is concerned with judging the worth of information (its currency and validity). Is it adequate, coherent and sufficient? Chapter 8 returns to the subject of evidence, an important sort of information.

Lastly, Gina refers to the *process* part of the skill. Reasoning is not only concerned with deciding what knowledge is appropriate, determining what is true, safe or effective and making judicious decisions; it is also concerned with how you plan your work. When a nurse gives an injection, he or she combines different sorts of knowledge to a clear purpose, but also determines the right order in which to proceed. For example, the nurse forewarns the patient about the planned injection, secures consent and then ensures a private environment to help protect the patient's dignity.

Activity 1.3 — *Critical thinking*

Explore with a chosen colleague an activity from your recent course learning to determine the different ways in which reasoning has had to work (deciding what you can claim, making decisions, reviewing knowledge and deciding on process). You are free to make your own selection, but possible activities include searching for references in the library, participating *continued ...* •

in the nursing shift handover report or perhaps practising a nursing technique after it has been demonstrated to you. Now, compare notes with your colleague on which of the skill components seemed toughest, and why. Appreciating what is toughest about critical thinking can help you to identify where you may have to concentrate harder, to check what you think you have understood or to ask questions of others.

In our experience, it is often the declarative component of a skill that seems hardest to students. There is sometimes no single 'right' answer. There are better answers and, to ascertain those, discussion and consultation with others is so important. That is why your course is likely to build in so much discussion time and why you are asked to 'think aloud'. All reasoning within a skill requires some effort, though.

No matter what part of your course you study, you will be engaged in critical thinking, combining and recombining the different components of nursing skill so you can proceed in ways that seem professional. Nursing practice has to be reasoned and the actions of the nurse reasonable. Indeed, in a court of law, judgements about whether a nurse's actions are negligent are based upon what a reasonable practitioner would do (Baylis, 2015). What Stewart and the others learn through their course is designed to enable them to work more safely, strategically, effectively (achieving required outcomes) and efficiently (using resources wisely).

Making critical thinking work for you

Having identified the different components of critical thinking only helps you so far. You need to consider how you might actually use critical thought to best effect and here aptitude, ability and

Student	Aptitude	Points made
Stewart	Asking questions	*If nurses don't ask questions about their work, they will never know what they don't know.*
Fatima	Discriminating	*Perhaps! But when you do know things you still have to decide what is relevant. We can't use every bit of information, we have to accept some information as being better for this situation.*
Raymet	Making arguments	*I wouldn't dismiss your points but here's a better one. Once you've decided that something is relevant you have to make arguments. I don't mean silly arguments, but the sort that help you defend what you think is best.*
Gina	Interpreting and speculating	*All worthy stuff ... but where is imagination in all this? The best nurse I ever saw was someone who kept imagining what could be different. She was always thinking about better solutions.*

Table 1.1: Critical thinking aptitudes

readiness to proceed come into play. For example, if a nurse fails to ask questions (an aptitude) and accepts the status quo, few improvements in practice can be expected. Quality of care may remain mediocre or even deteriorate further. Doing the same thing in the same way is unlikely to produce change.

Let's return again to the four nurses. In Table 1.1, the colleagues each suggest an aptitude that they think is important to the successful nurse. All of the aptitudes within this table have a justifiable role in critical thinking. It is significant that we think of these as aptitudes. Aptitudes are something that you probably have already, but in nursing they need to be developed further and to a very high degree. Some people argue better than others; they are persuasive and able to convey their thinking clearly. Others are more imaginative and comfortable speculating about how nursing care could be. They speculate in safe places, away from the bedside, and discuss ideas with patients that sometimes transform the way in which care is delivered.

Activity 1.4   *Critical thinking*

Study Table 1.1 and decide how important you rate the aptitude suggested by each of the student nurses (of great importance, of some importance, neither important nor unimportant, of little importance, of no importance). Write down a short rationale for each of your decisions, relating those to nursing as you understand it today.

We now examine each aptitude in more depth.

Asking questions

Asking questions is certainly important, but individuals vary in their level of confidence. Perhaps you worry that asking questions suggests an uncomfortable level of ignorance or gaps in your knowledge. Asking questions, though, and especially when working with professional colleagues, is at the heart of health care. For example, questions are frequently used to clarify the best care options and, at best, these involve patients in decisions made. All members of the team offer questions – ones that are designed to examine alternative explanations of what has been learned and what might resolve a problem in the future. Sometimes the more naive question is the one that transforms the team's understanding of a clinical situation. You may hear nurse mentors rehearsing questions aloud as an aid to planning or adjusting care. 'These are some questions that I would ask myself at this stage about educating patients,' they might say. What does the patient need to do now? When are they in the right position to start mobilising? In Part 3 of this book we turn to the business of expressing critical thinking, and one of the things that distinguishes the level of your critical thinking in coursework is the questions that you choose to explore. If you rely on set questions, those that do not take account of prevailing healthcare circumstances, those that are less nuanced, then your writing might be judged as sound but not especially critical. You are working with a formula for what might be asked, and that might mean that you miss important issues to explore.

You can improve your question asking by:

- Deciding what it is exactly that you need to know, being precise as regards what you ask about. Asking what are the possible side effects of a named cancer chemotherapy drug is much better than asking about them collectively. Different drugs may produce different side effects.

- Formulating your question in a way that establishes your focus of interest. It often helps for example to link your question to a point just taught; this will help the tutor understand the context of your question. It may reassure them that you have a sincere interest in what they have argued.

- Jotting down your question before you ask it. This is important in lectures and conference sessions where your anxiety at asking a question might otherwise mean the question is fumbled.

- Deciding whether you want to ask a closed or an open question. A closed question is one that prompts a yes or no answer. For example, 'Am I correct in understanding that you think patients have a duty to collaborate on care planning?' An open question is one that prompts a more expansive answer from the other person. 'Can you explain why you think patients should collaborate with the nurse on care planning?'

Discriminating

There comes a stage where we have to discriminate between what is relevant and irrelevant, and what is true and what is false. Discrimination involves weighing information and determining what enables us to make arguments, such that might be supported by others. One example of discrimination in action is where a nurse searches for empirical evidence to support a given practice. The nurse reasons that the information supplied through research studies is superior to that derived from anecdote, at least where the design of research has been rigorous and clearly described. If you are judging the claims made by others, one way of showing discrimination is to ponder the circumstances or conditions under which an argument might be false. 'Under what conditions might it not be advantageous for the patient to remain in their own home to receive nursing care?' is an example of a question that might be used. Most claims can be falsified under one condition or another, so you will quickly realise that health care involves probabilities. What is probably true? What can probably be supported as a case?

Hammond (1978, 1996, 2007) describes a cognitive continuum of reasoning. At one extreme is the scientific experiment, which is carefully controlled but, of course, is not necessarily practical to replicate in nursing practice. At the other extreme is what is called 'weak quasi-rational thought', where the nurse works more with intuition. Some of your first discrimination reasoning might be associated with determining whether relevant evidence exists in the first place. After that, there is the matter of deciding whether the evidence is valid and reliable, and whether it fits with practice requirements. In Chapter 8, we explain how reasoning and evidence are both affected by paradigms – accepted ways of understanding and evaluating the world around us. There may be no single best way of reasoning, only the best way to deal with the sort of information encountered.

We might imagine a mentor weighing up the case made by researchers in an article she has read. The article describes a study of how patients with diabetes were taught to care for themselves. The mentor might debate the following:

- Is what the authors claim true?

- Are there any competing explanations for this?

- Is the information coherent and its origins appropriately explained?

Showing appropriate discrimination in your reasoning will be important in your coursework. You will need to demonstrate that you have considered possible explanations of what you see or hear, and that you then determine what you need to consider before you elect a particular course of action. In Part 3 of this book, we discuss different levels of critical thinking in your writing, and one of the markers of higher level critical thinking is that not only can you identify what must be discriminated between (the competing explanations) but you can reason why one explanation seems better than another. Where writing shows little or no recognition of competing explanations, it might be described as uncritical or even opinionated. Only one explanation has been considered and that one is counted as adequate without much further thought.

Making arguments

Arguments are formulated about a variety of things: what should be done next; what this literature suggests is valuable; what constitutes compassionate care. Arguments are necessary, as they explain the basis of nursing in action and why we are working to the goals that we have. An argument is made up of premises (that is, the things that we accept as fact or likely to be true) and a conclusion, which we believe follows from the premises that we have presented (Swatridge, 2014). The connection between premise and conclusion is supported by observations or other evidence, perhaps from research. So, for example, we might make an argument about patient anxiety and how it interferes with collaborative care planning. Our conclusion might be that we must adequately attend to expressed patient anxiety in order to secure their cooperation in care planning. The premises mustered to support such a conclusion are drawn from different places. We might point to teaching received on perception and attention span. Patients cannot cooperate if they are distracted by anxiety. To connect the conclusion to the premise we muster evidence: evidence drawn from experience of patients and their level of care planning cooperation, and perhaps also from research on what patients understand about collaborative care planning when they begin working with the nurse. As can be seen in later chapters, arguments are central to successful analytical essays and your ability to convince others within these. Arguments need to be measured, calm and well considered. Those that simply appeal to emotion will not help the nurse to make a case. Assignment answers that are judged as showing more critical thinking are usually those that have clear and well-rounded arguments, and that are strongly associated with paragraphs that focus clearly on a topic, that muster evidence and then lead the reader through what the argument is and why it is plausible. We return to this again in Part 3 of the book.

Our example mentor above might accept that the research report shared was indeed relevant to our chosen practice setting, and that the design of the study was rigorous. The researchers have shown all their 'workings out' along the way. However, she might then argue that, because there has been a local policy change, only part of the evidence can be incorporated in future care delivered. Successful arguments (van den Brink-Budgen, 2010):

- have a clear focus (are sure what they are about);
- indicate what is preferred or recommended, or what cannot yet be determined (your case);
- provide a rationale for why the chosen case is made.

In nursing, the rationale for an argument may be based on evidence but it might also be based on moral justice (Larchman, 2012). Some arguments are made on ethical grounds, regarding what *should* be done. In clinical practice, a wide variety of factors impinge upon arguments made, including those relating to ethical best practice, what will have the greatest therapeutic effect, what can or should be afforded and what must be prioritised when competing demands arise and health-care resources are necessarily limited. Uncomfortable as it may be, nurses have to make arguments based upon moral justice, especially in circumstances where they believe that the rights of patients are under threat (Game, 2014). As a nurse, you will sometimes need to be the advocate for patients and their rights, as has been highlighted within reports on shortfalls in healthcare service delivery (Francis, 2013). Compassionate and caring nurses sometimes need to confront the arguments of others, asserting a case that protects the patient and sustains best standards of nursing care.

A good way to strengthen your arguments within a debate is to show that you have carefully considered alternative arguments, other ways to see the situation. You then reject other arguments by offering a rationale regarding why they are not valid, relevant or supportable given the context in which care is delivered.

Activity 1.5   *Group work*

Discuss with your colleagues the following argument, to decide whether it is supportable. You might, for example, ask the questions:

'What would need to be evident for this argument to be valid?'

'What would need to apply if this argument was to be considered relevant?'

'Are there any points, experiences or observations that might support other arguments?'

Argument

Nurses facilitate patient rehabilitation by teaching the patient skills, monitoring and correcting their performance of the skills and rewarding them with verbal encouragement.

Whole books on the philosophy of reasoning and rhetoric are available and we suggest further resources at the end of this chapter. Very simply, however, each of the following might have fairly been part of your deliberations in Activity 1.5.

- Observations of whether in fact nurses have been involved in teaching work of this kind (the argument asserts a fact, rather than a value, nurses *should* facilitate patient rehabilitation).
- Deliberation of whether this is the sole or the primary way in which rehabilitation is facilitated.

- Consideration as to whether patients are ready, willing and able to act as learners (teaching assumes some degree of cooperation).

- Discussions regarding whether nurses are equipped to teach, monitor, assess and correct the performance of the skill.

If the nurse never has the time, confidence or training to engage in teaching work of this kind, then the argument is irrelevant. It remains a theoretical point, one perhaps to which nurses should subscribe. Much of your learning as you move back and forth between campus and clinical practice relates to the formulation and examination of arguments, including those relating to what works in practice.

Interpreting and speculating

Interpreting involves making sense of that which is encountered. A variety of stimuli are received by the nurse (e.g., auditory – what patients or others say; visual – how patients look; olfactory – whether a wound smells; touch – whether the patient feels hot) and these are converted into perceptions when the nurse combines stimuli with past experience (memory). Successful interpretation then relies upon being alert to all the possible stimuli, and then understanding how these can be combined to determine what is happening (e.g. Bergevin, 2014; Lowth, 2014). Sometimes conflicting stimuli will be encountered that make it harder for the nurse to understand what is happening (e.g., signs and symptoms of illness that signal several different possible diseases). Nurses develop their interpretation skills as experience accumulates and more examples of what happened, what followed and what was important are then understood. Writing about the importance of experience in learning, Benner (2001) describes how practice is initially rule-governed but is later based on principles of best practice. This transition is supported by a careful consideration of perceptions – what we believe we have witnessed.

We have left speculation until last, and consider it extremely important. Successful nursing relies in significant part on nurses 'thinking outside the box', daring to consider options or solutions that are unfamiliar. Creativity and imagination therefore form a valuable part of critical thinking and one that can help nurses improve the lot of patients.

Gina talks about her clinical mentor:

My mentor pulled all the information together about teaching the diabetic patients and quickly realised that, with the staff available, they couldn't do it in the old familiar way. That was when she suggested that they should teach patients in groups and organise the sessions so the patients helped one another out. As the patients assisted one another, my mentor watched them and decided who understood the insulin treatment best.

A readiness to speculate, about what is problematic or what could be done better or differently to make the best use of finite resources and expertise available, is often at the heart of high-quality health care and highly rated coursework assignments. Even when others prefer to work with the familiar, the status quo, it is incumbent upon nurses to examine what is being done and what could be done to further improve the care of patients. Wild speculation, that which does not adequately assess healthcare risks, that which has no regard for equity of care to a group of patients as well as the individual, that which is naive about healthcare resources, is to be avoided. But you should dare to think differently too, to imagine other ways of doing things. Do not assume that the old ways are always the best, or that others have always spotted changing circumstances – that which might mandate a new approach to nursing care, a new opportunity.

How can we reason better?

However appealing it seems to place the above aptitudes in a set sequence and to say that this is the best or right way to reason, we have to acknowledge that critical thinking is a little less formulaic than this. Nurses often start by asking questions, but they could also start by preparing arguments before testing these out against what they read or see. We call tentative arguments of this kind 'working hypotheses' – draft explanations of what we think is happening and what will happen next. Reasoning therefore seems to work in two ways and sometimes in parallel.

- **Deductively**: we test working hypotheses to see whether what we predict is, in fact, the case (for example, the nurse has an idea regarding how best to persuade a patient to give up cigarettes and tries that out in practice).

- **Inductively**: we continue gathering information in order to formulate theories and explanations of what is happening (for example, the nurse observes when the patient seems most in need of a cigarette each day to decide what sustains their smoking habit; the nurse then prepares a working theory regarding what might help them to counter that, and what will help them to give up cigarettes).

Activity 1.6   *Group work*

This group exercise is designed to help you with the terms thinking *inductively* and *deductively*. To help check your understanding of these terms, pair up with a colleague and ask your associate to first offer a theory to explain what makes it easier to help a patient to rehabilitate (thinking inductively). Perhaps they refer to experiences of delivering care to one or more patients. You are making theory from experience.

Next, report to your colleague what you have read about the nursing process, about the philosophy of nursing, that should help you to support patient rehabilitation in an individualised way (deductive reasoning). You are working from theory towards experience.

Which of these two sorts of thinking seemed most comfortable and why? Both are needed in nursing, although some students are surprised by the importance of inductive learning. Their past experience in school or college may have emphasised the importance of learning from theory, rather than theorising.

Critical thinking is, in many instances, like working on a jigsaw puzzle. We attend to different parts of the problem or need, making progress in one area because this seems necessary now. Problem-based learning courses emphasise exactly this process (Pilcher, 2014). Students are presented with outline case studies and search for further information in order to plan care. The process of learning to make sense of ambiguous situations is at the centre of study and replicates the conditions that are met in practice.

Working on your aptitudes enables you to develop progressively more sophisticated approaches to critical thinking. Moon (2008) summarises these as part of her wide-ranging discussion on ways of thinking about knowledge. Instead of seeing situations in deceptively simplistic terms, the thinker learns to explore the complexity of healthcare situations. The more sophisticated our reasoning, the more flexible and comfortable we become as we consider each problem, challenge or need in turn. We become better at making sense of what is happening, identifying what could happen next and how we might then best proceed.

Activity 1.7 — *Decision making*

Look now at the ways of reasoning described in Table 1.2 and decide which you think are the more sophisticated forms of reasoning and which are the least sophisticated. Decide for yourself if you employ one of these approaches more than others.

Reasoning approach	Description
Contextual knowing	We rely strongly on contexts to determine what we focus upon and accept as important and valuable. For example, we might suggest that the circumstances of a family of a dying patient strongly influence how they cope with news that the illness is incurable.
Independent knowing	So much knowledge is constructed by people. For example, a dental appointment is understood (as good or bad) with regard to our previous experiences of dental treatment. So we search experience to suggest clues on how to think about things and then take up our position on that subject.
Transitional knowing	Reasoning involves living with doubts, about what is true, best, defensible or important. We learn to wait and see and accept that right now several explanations of the situation might be supportable.
Silent absorption	Individuals absorb and appreciate a growing volume of information, contemplating the same without necessarily venturing an opinion. For example, a student attends a series of lectures on physiology, venturing no opinion on what is discussed there until all the important facts are to hand.
Absolute knowing	We search for what is right or wrong, making clear distinctions – that which is fact and that which is not. We search for the definitive answer that properly supports care decisions.

Table 1.2: Ways of reasoning

Debate continues about what represents more or less sophisticated forms of reasoning. Nursing demands different forms of reasoning at different times but, here, we venture the following. The least sophisticated forms of reasoning are what Baxter-Magolda (1992) calls *absolute*. At this level, the individual is unable to see the different nuances of a situation or to accept that a range of possible perspectives could be taken on a subject. The thinker looks for certainty and only feels secure when matters have been decisively concluded: 'this is right; that is wrong; this is what we believe; this is what we don't believe'. If you are prone to thinking in this way, you might note how often you ask the tutor or your practice mentor to be expert, to define what is 'correct'. While an absolute might be expected with regard to some areas of work, for example the right drug to use in an emergency, it is not something that is possible or even desirable in many other situations (e.g., finding the right ways to demonstrate that we are listening). We need to be more flexible in our approach. Absolute thinking is a common way of reasoning, especially at the start of a university education.

We have placed *silent absorption* next, at least where the individual feels incapable of comprehending what the important issues are. The thinker waits, soaking up more and more information in the hope that reasoning will be assisted by the accumulation of knowledge. In practice, this does not always work out, even though it may have been your tried and tested way of reasoning. More information does not always lead to clarity and there is a need to ask questions and discuss ideas if we are to develop confidence in our reasoning.

We suggest that *transitional thinking* comes next: the thinker is ready to live with the uncertainties of knowledge, but is ready, as well, to question as opportunities present. You will need to reason in this way, accepting that, in some clinical contexts, and for the time being, not all can be understood about a situation. Insights emerge from what is experienced and discussed and, in the meantime, it is necessary to remain alert to what experience or a carefully selected question can assist you with. For example, this happens as we monitor a developing illness in a patient and determine how best to modify treatment, controlling body temperature or adjusting fluid balance.

Contextual thinking is even more sophisticated and suggests that the thinker understands that there are lots of different truths in the world and what works in one context does not work in another. This is not to suggest that you have no principles or standards and that 'anything goes' within nursing. Principles and safe practice are important, but there may well be different ways of doing things within those parameters. A good example of this working well is where nurses explore with patients the nature of dignity. What represents dignified care can vary widely and takes into account patient expectations, lifestyle and custom (Manookian et al., 2014).

Independent thinking is arguably the most sophisticated form of reasoning and one that helps you to become more innovative over time. At this level, you allow others to adopt their own position and to develop arguments in support of the same, while you build your own case about the subject in hand. You carefully search what there is to support your own position, stand ready to change it if others can persuade you, and treat all discussion in a thoughtful and enquiring way. An example of this might be where the nurse adopts a clear and defensible stance associated with an extended role (practice beyond the normal job remit), exploring its benefits in health care, but also considering what might be lost if new duties are taken on (Joel, 2009).

As you review your answers to Activity 1.7, do not be alarmed if you thought that your own thinking was near the bottom of this hierarchy. Students frequently need to work from the bottom. Moving from more familiar ways of reasoning to those that involve greater uncertainty and challenge means that you have to move out of your comfort zone. Excellent tutors are adept at helping students to do this, respecting their anxieties, but always searching for better ways to help them explore nursing. This is one of the key reasons why your course is likely to involve different sorts of learning activity (e.g., lectures, discussion groups, demonstrations, role play). Each, in some regard, practises you in different forms of reasoning and promotes what you will need to demonstrate in order to be a successful practitioner.

Chapter summary

We have introduced you to basic ideas about critical thinking and explained that it is a process, involving the gathering, receiving and processing of information in order to understand the world around you. It is important in nursing for a number of reasons: those associated with safety, with creativity, with problem solving and the management of a great deal of uncertainty that often attends patients and their needs. Nurses need to be able to declare what they believe to be true and trustworthy, as the basis for subsequent action. Equally important is a grasp of process – how care is delivered, what treatment works and why. Reasoning in this sense guides the nurse in a series of daily activities that help patients with their needs.

Another component of reasoning that makes it important is decision making – deciding what to do next when nurses and colleagues have incomplete information. Knowledge accumulation and application are important. Nurses have to combine a lot of theoretical knowledge and know when to apply it, and reasoning is central to this work.

For reasoning to work in practice, though, and for the component parts of this skill to work together, nurses must develop certain aptitudes. These include asking questions, making arguments, speculating and discriminating. It is highly likely that there remains considerable scope for you to develop these further during the course of your studies. Rest assured, it is quite natural for students to have anxieties about these and tutors understand this. Part 2 of this book returns to many of these matters afresh.

Finally, we have briefly explored ways in which we might recognise more sophisticated forms of reasoning. Some areas of nursing work will require these; for instance with regard to professional ethics, innovation in practice or the development of care philosophies that show how we work best with patients. Studying this material should have helped you to decide where your own reasoning has progressed to so far and to identify when it is improving in the future. Completion of the chapter activities will have afforded you the opportunity to do several things, including the examination of arguments and identification of what within your reasoning is already well developed.

Further reading

Ellis, P (2013) *Evidence-Based Practice in Nursing*, 2nd ed. London: Sage/Learning Matters.

Peter Ellis and co-authors provide a tour of the different sorts of evidence, indicating the critical thinking required in order to evaluate each. Especially useful is Chapter 1, which explores the critical thinking disposition to utilise evidence and engage in evidence-based practice.

Moon, J (2008) *Critical Thinking: An exploration of theory and practice.* Abingdon: Routledge.

This demanding but valuable book remains one of the most insightful discussions of what critical thinking entails. Moon catalogues why critical thinking is hard to describe and in Chapter 6 discusses 'academic assertiveness', something that is encouraged among nurse learners.

Standing, M (2014) *Clinical Judgement and Decision Making for Nursing Students*, 2nd ed. London: Sage/Learning Matters.

Mooi Standing details what underpins so much of clinical decision making: the ways in which critical judgements are made in practice. This book provides an important illustration of applied critical thinking, drawing on ethics and evidence as well as experience.

Swatridge, C (2014) *Oxford Guide to Effective Argument and Critical Thinking.* Oxford: Oxford University Press.

Swatridge takes a classical approach to the study of reasoning, the development of arguments, the exploration of inferences and the examination of that which seems plausible. While this book is not written specifically for healthcare professionals, the principles contained here still hold good. It is a particularly valuable book if you feel committed to a particular healthcare cause and wish to examine the competing arguments in some depth.

Useful websites

Note: website material is subject to change or removal at short notice. The following is only indicative of valuable content.

www.Wikihow.com/Make-a-Logical-Argument

This simple three-step guide on the formation of arguments will assist you to understand what is necessary as you try to make your thinking more critical. Start by knowing your premises, what you accept as facts. Then structure your argument, show how the premise is supported by observations or data and then proceed to the conclusion of it (stating what you deduce). Finally, avoid some classic fallacies of argument formation.

https://danielmiessler.com/blog/how-to-build-a-strong-argument

This blog written by Miessler in 2009 adds more information about the differences between deductive and inductive reasoning. It also introduces you gently to classical reasoning as employed in philosophy.

www.sussex.ac.uk/s3/?id=87-Critical_thinking:s3:University_of_Sussex

Most universities have something to offer on critical thinking and its importance in academic work, often located in the website as 'study support'. It is a good idea also to check out resources where you study. This example, from the University of Sussex, is recommended because it highlights the culture of critical analysis expected of students at university. Look at the student video clips to hear how they are using critical thinking in their courses.

www.prepareforsuccess.org.uk/critical_thinking.html

We like the interactive nature of the activities included here and believe that you should be able to complete them after working through this chapter. The site provides feedback against which you can compare the answers you type into the screen.

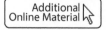
Additional Online Material

For examples of analytical essays and other useful material, please visit the companion website at **www.sagepub.co.uk/price_harrington**

Chapter 2
Reflecting

Chapter aims

After reading this chapter, you will be able to:

- define reflection, indicating how a stated purpose can help make reflections more critical;
- distinguish the differences between reflecting in practice and on practice, detailing why they are different from one another;
- identify six reasons why reflection is important in nursing, noting those that appear in most frequent use;
- discuss the best principles of reflection, identifying how you will proceed in the future;
- explain why it is important to ascertain course expectations associated with frameworks for reflection, and whether reflection should be practised at both the intimate and the skill review level.

Introduction

Nursing courses are strongly associated with the skill of reflection and for good reasons. However, reflection is a skill we have all engaged in and all use on a regular basis, one that is facilitated by soap operas or reality shows we see on television. What delights us there is the opportunity to debate what was said and done, and what might have been said or done as an alternative. Behaviour was 'wise', 'foolish', 'typical of that character' or 'critical to what happened next'. We are all armchair experts.

In this chapter, we start with some distinctions between reflecting on the here and now, and on what has gone before. This is an excellent way to focus our attention on reflection, because we believe you will quickly note some practical differences between the two, and this will help you to discover just how important reflection can be. Next, we share our own definition of reflection and help you to identify why it is distinct from other forms of critical thinking. While reflection has classically centred on the individual care episode, we suggest that it needs to connect onwards to an understanding of care relationships, to the narratives and discourses that are important there (Price, 2011a). Reflection focuses on experience and admits feelings into the equation.

We proceed then to a review of why reflection is so essential in nursing and why it is emphasised within your nursing course. Particular emphasis is placed on the development of empathy, an ability to imagine the feelings and needs of others while still respecting our own professional role. Empathy is important if the nurse is to meet several of the six Cs (Department of Health and NHS Commissioning Board, 2012). Care, compassion, successful communication and commitment all start with a clear understanding about how others experience nursing care. We need to imagine how our practice impinges on others. Finally, the chapter explores some of the best principles of reflection which you will need to take into account as you reflect alongside your course studies.

Activity 2.1   *Reflection*

Consider this argument: 'It is easier to reflect after the event rather than during it.'

- Do you support this argument?
- What premises (that which we already accept as fact) underpin your position on the argument?
- What evidence (including that from experience) can you identify which either supports or challenges the argument?

Schön (1987) believes reflecting on action is different from reflecting in action. If we reflect on the event as it unfolds, we have none of the benefits of calm introspection and time to consider at leisure the different options available to us. Against that, if we reflect long after the event, it is likely that memory may play tricks on us and we may remember certain features of the event better than others. Reflecting in practice involves 'thinking on our feet' (Koharchik et al., 2015). We have to attend very quickly to what others say or do and accommodate the feelings that quickly well up inside us as we deal with the events as they unfold. We cannot pause the action in order to produce the sage-like response that we would love to deliver. Reflecting in action is in some sense rather 'raw', but perhaps all the more vivid for that. We can illustrate that with two short excerpts of reflection from an experienced staff nurse called Lauren. In the first extract, Lauren is reflecting in action and in the second she reflects on action. It is important to note that in-action reflections are usually unspoken. Speaking aloud our thoughts could prove problematic in many clinical settings.

In the following case study, Lauren has encountered a potentially aggressive relative.

Case study: Reflection in action and reflecting on practice

Reflecting in action

Is this man going to hit me ... he seems really angry? What does he want? I need to say something, do something that shows him I respect his concerns. I need to suggest something. I know, I'll suggest we talk in the relatives' room, but leaving the door open in case I need assistance. That shows I will give him time to tell me what worries him, and I'll remain safe! Yes, that seems to have worked, he is agreeing to accompany me. But he's still talking as we go – he's like a pressure cooker and I'm worried about how that will seem to the other relatives on the ward ...

Reflecting on practice

The relative had suffered a major shock. He thought he had nearly a week to prepare for his wife to come home and here she was ready to be discharged that afternoon! No wonder he was fuming. We were meeting our needs to make a bed available for someone else and foisting the patient back into his care at short notice. Colleagues could see his wife required some more rehabilitation at home, so this was going to be a significant responsibility for him.

The above excerpts show just how different reflecting seems at these points. Notice the staccato way in which thoughts emerge when reflecting in action. There is an urgent search for meaning. Lauren has to work with her perceptions of what the relative is feeling, as well as her own experiences of a confrontation. The reflections on action are evaluative and confident, and indicate considerable empathy for the man. Lauren can assert a great deal more about the origins of the problem. The important point here is that reflecting in action is necessarily less considered, less perfect than that which is possible afterwards. It can be very hard to attend to your feelings, thoughts and next actions while also trying to understand the behaviour of someone else.

In your nursing course, you will be asked to prepare reflective practice coursework. Demonstrating your powers of reflection is important. There are different levels of reflection, however, something we discuss further in the next chapter of this book. What is usually sought is critical reflection: harder to achieve if you reflect in practice. Objective structured clinical examinations and bedside observation examinations simulate, to differing degrees, reflection in action (Martensson and Lofmark, 2013), but most assessment invites you to reflect on practice in retrospect. Critical reflection requires you to take an overview and understand how your own values, beliefs and goals affect the way in which you approach patients and how that in turn interacts with how they feel and what they might wish to achieve. It is much harder to 'see the bigger picture' if you are in the midst of healthcare events.

In your course, the opportunities to reflect on practice may be legion. You will be asked to write reflective essays, and to develop case studies which explore the quality of care delivered to patients. The very act of recording reflections in a written account makes them retrospective in act (we think faster than we can write). Opportunities to reflect in action and with support are much rarer. If you are fortunate, they occur with an experienced practical skills teacher or clinical mentor, who helps you to rehearse aloud your thinking within a psychologically safe environment, where a reflective account does not alarm patients (Lovatt, 2014).

As you think about reflecting in and on action, it is valuable to understand what you are trying to do. First, you encounter behaviour of others – this may take the form of action (a hug, a shake of the fist, a smile) – and try to interpret that. But you also listen to an *account* of their experiences, feelings or attitudes ('I'm livid my wife has to come home from hospital without any preparation at all!'). Lying beneath that account, and either more or less coherently expressed, there may be a *narrative* – an underlying story the individual uses to make sense of what is happening and what they are trying to accomplish (Price, 2011b). In this instance, the narrative might relate to buying more discharge preparation time, or securing some think time to understand what caring for his wife will now involve. The whole encounter, though, may be part of a bigger storyline – a *discourse*, which is something that helps to explain what is under way. The obvious discourse here concerns discharge planning and lay care liaison (process and technique). But it might also be about

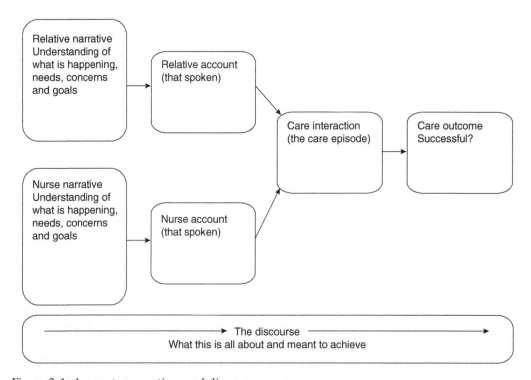

Figure 2.1: Accounts, narratives and discourses

managing pressures on bed occupancy, or the need to prompt relatives to become active lay carers when this was not a part of their past role. Discourses must usually take account of your goals, your values and attitudes as well. When encountering an aggressive patient, you will do so with a number of attitudes already developed. It is unreasonable to assault a nurse; we are caring staff. But angry people do not behave rationally, so a primary goal is to stay safe. What I really want to achieve here is a win–win situation – one where the relative feels respected and we can find a solution to the patient discharge from hospital problem. Stakeholders within a discourse might disagree vehemently about what is under way and what should happen. Figure 2.1 illustrates how these elements might fit together.

Reflecting in action, then, is really rather taxing. We respond to and share accounts about what is going on, but have some awareness, too, of what we want to achieve, our agenda and the explanation of events as we think of these (our narrative). We have too, if acting professionally, a concern for the needs of others – their underlying narrative. We try to understand that in the process of care giving. But we also work with a discourse, one that might have been taught within your course ('delivering individualised care') or required as part of organisational policy (managing bed occupancy).

Activity 2.2   *Reflection*

Return now to your responses to Activity 2.1 and determine whether what you have learned about accounts, narratives and discourses has helped you to further explain the differences between reflecting in and on action. Are there some circumstances where revisiting the attitudes, beliefs and values you hold, those exposed by care situations, might seem difficult to evaluate as part of reflection in practice? What happens, for instance, if you deal with patients who have different beliefs, values and lifestyles to your own? Existentialist philosophers emphasise the challenge of making sense of life and our relationships. Some of our values and beliefs have been *tacit*; that is, unconsidered until now and taken for granted (Eriksen et al., 2014). Then ponder the value of reflection on action, in retrospect. Does this provide better opportunities to reconsider your values and beliefs, perhaps those exercised by a series of different care encounters?

Defining reflection

The above early distinction between reflecting in practice and on practice serves us well, as we explore next the definition of reflection used within this book. Reflection is a skill used in two contexts – during events and after them. We think of reflection as a subset skill of critical thinking and one used in close association with experience. It involves the use of decision making (reflecting in action) and evaluation (reflecting on action). In both cases, we are making sense of events around us and trying to use our personal aptitudes in order to work in ways that seem more sensitive and successful. For example, to reflect in action, it is important that we are able to think of our own actions as we might when watching an actor on stage. We have to consider not only what happened and how we felt, but also what our own motives or goals might have been for that situation (Howatson-Jones, 2016).

To take the case of Lauren, there is a need to speculate about how we can best assist this angry relative to express his concerns in a way that limits the risk of violence. This aptitude is called metacognition (Norris and Gimber, 2013). It is the process of considering our own motives and actions as they work in concert with those of others involved in an event. Another important aptitude associated with reflection (especially on action) is empathy. We need to be able to appreciate the actions of others in context and with reference to circumstances that brought the event about (Atherton and Kyle, 2015).

Reflection, then, is:

> *a process whereby experience is examined in ways that give meaning to interaction. We might examine the experience in real time or in retrospect. Because experience engages the emotions as well as reasoning, reflection needs to take account of the feelings engendered within an interaction and to allow that perceptions (how we interpret matters) may sometimes prove erroneous. While reflection is most closely associated with human interactions and especially clinical events, it is not limited to these. We may, for instance, reflect upon the written accounts of experiences, such as those shared by dying patients. Reflection may be used in the service of different nursing goals – those that are designed to tell us something about how we think, what we value, and with regard to ways in which practice could be improved.*

Why reflecting is important

Figure 2.2 represents some of the reasons why reflection is so important in nursing. Just how apparent these are depends in part on how far you have progressed through your course of study.

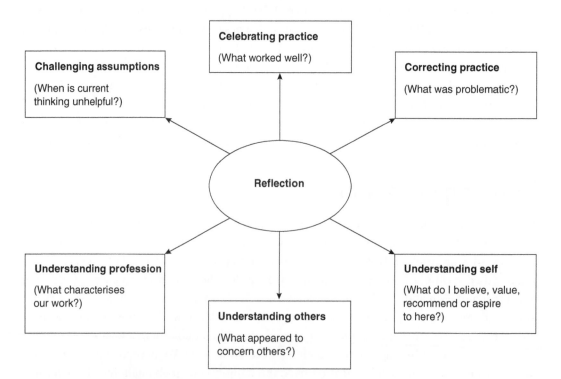

Figure 2.2: Why reflection is important in nursing

Some of the rationale for reflection only becomes apparent as you study within different learning environments and deal with different subjects within the curriculum.

***

Annotate Figure 2.2 with a score in each box to indicate how frequently you have observed reflection being used to that purpose in your course so far. If, for example, it is used very frequently indeed score it 3, if it is used regularly score it 2, if it is used only occasionally score it 1, and if you have never seen it used for that purpose score it 0. Date these scores, so you can return to this activity later to see whether these have changed as your experience grows. Consider next whether reflection is primarily seen as a corrective tool or one that liberates nursing.

As this is a personal observation activity we don't provide answers of our own, but read on now to explore further the purposes of reflection in nursing.

***

Celebrating practice

Reflection on action can be put to excellent use to celebrate practice that is successful and which exceeds the expectations we have of it. It is not enough for nurses to simply pat themselves on the back for a job well done. We need to understand how we brought about the desirable outcomes (Balasubramanian et al., 2010). Nurses need to know how to replicate successful care and perhaps then to transfer that to other situations where problems can be solved (e.g. Long et al., 2014). As you think about reflection used for this purpose, it is necessary to be clear about the criteria used to define success. Do we mean more effective care (greater impact), more efficient care (better use of resources), more sensitive care (working with the needs of patients) or more collegiate care (working better with other professions)? There are six C questions to which you might refer when defining why nursing is timely, successful and empathetic. Was it caring (working closely with patient needs), was it compassionate (responsive to the concerns of patients and their hurt, loss or anxiety), was it competent (demonstrating safe and skilful nursing work done)? Was the practice an example of good communication (we need to work with other professionals as well as patients and relatives)? Did it exhibit courage? There are times when a nurse must act as an advocate of the patient, especially if poor or negligent practice is witnessed. Did the practice show due commitment, both to the patient and to the high standards of service, those typically espoused in the mission statement of a healthcare organisation or team? (Department of Health and NHS Commissioning Board, 2012).

While much nursing care relates to meeting measurable targets, working in concert with others to sustain healthcare protocols, you should not lose sight of the fact that, of all healthcare professions, nurses are arguably among the most empathetic. Our mission is to help others to deal with the experience of illness, injury or disability as well as the problems themselves. To be empathetic is to understand how others process their experiences, how they make sense of what is happening. With this in mind, much of what is successful in nursing is not easily understood in statistical or target terms. Instead, we focus carefully on patient feedback, the testimony shared on how care felt. Reflection is an excellent means of exploring such empathy. For example, when reviewing letters of thanks, what are the recurring satisfaction themes reported? What do patients really notice and value?

Correcting practice

Reflection is frequently used to determine what went wrong and what was problematic. *In extremis* it may be used to determine who we believe was to blame for untoward events. Reflection is employed, for instance, as part of a root cause analysis (searching for the origins of a problem) in cases where there are shortfalls in practice or where there has been a near miss (e.g., associated with a drug error). Root cause analysis gives focus to reflection and sharpens critical awareness of what went wrong (Carter et al., 2014). Reflecting in this way, on what was problematic or erroneous, is taxing. It is emotionally difficult to confront what we believe were our mistakes, and what we might have done better or differently. It becomes more problematic within a blame culture, such as in health care, where performances are meant to be faultless.

Reflecting on what seems problematic is often made easier where a mentor is available to assist you. This individual explores with you your perceptions of events and helps you to examine the conclusions you reach. How big a problem was this? Why did it occur? What were my options? What decisions were important here? What are the pluses as well as the minuses of the course of action that I chose?

Understanding self

Authors vary on the extent to which they think reflection should be used to understand ourselves (Bulman and Schutz, 2008; Craig, 2009). In some areas of nursing (e.g., mental health or palliative care) an understanding of our motives, values and personality is especially important because we use the self to therapeutic purpose. Our ability to share personal insights, or to imagine how others feel, may be critical (Olsen, 2013). Instead of seeing the nurse as someone who musters and applies skills, the nurse is conceived as someone who uses his or her personality as part of therapy. The ability to empathise, for example, becomes integral to entering the world of the patient and their anxieties, but one that must be managed with a certain detachment as well if professional judgements are then to remain sound. A successful nurse builds an excellent rapport with patients and empathises with some of their concerns, but also manages to adopt a position where they can later challenge some of the patients' unhelpful beliefs.

These are important points and may be the focus for some of your concerns as well as some of your later nursing achievements. If you think of nursing in craft terms, your emphasis is likely to be on skills and the ways these are selected and applied. For example, with regard to interpersonal relationships with patients, your reflections may focus on techniques, such as listening or clarifying options open to the patient. If, though, you think of nursing in much more aesthetic terms, you are likely to feel more comfortable reflecting on your values and beliefs, precisely because you see these as a means to deliver the best care. In recent years, and under considerable healthcare service pressures, the values of nurses have come under increasing scrutiny. Shortfalls in care at Mid-Staffordshire Hospital NHS Trust have meant that nurses must now reassure the public of their professional values and intent (Francis, 2013). It is no longer taken for granted that nurses have a vocation and will instinctively do the right thing. For that reason, we are likely to see more and more coursework assessment relating to whether nurses are ready to explore their values and beliefs and to address personal attitudes that might in some sense seem less appropriate.

What is clear is that, within the coursework you produce, you must prove that you can be introspective. It is not enough to take things for granted and assume that a particular course of action is intrinsically correct. Successful and sensitive nursing care is nuanced; it fits with the circumstances of the care environment. You will then have to revisit those circumstances and what you were trying to do if you are to claim within your work that you are being critically reflective. We discuss this further in Part 3, where we look at examples of reflective practice writing.

Understanding others

Much of nursing is concerned with assisting others. Person-centred care is based upon the premise that we can successfully ascertain the patient's needs and aspirations, before taking these into account as part of the care we agree (Karlsson et al., 2014). If we are to practise sensitively, to respect cultural diversity, the different ways in which people live and manage health, illness and treatment, then we must understand people and their background. There are some problems, though, with using reflection to understand others; chief among these is what we might call the 'common sense' fallacy. We might take it as a given that people in a particular situation (e.g., when suffering pain) will wish to proceed as we would (to have that pain alleviated). We start to use our preferences and wishes in such situations as something we believe that others will aspire to as well. In reality, not all patients do aspire to alleviate all of their pain; indeed, some may refuse pain relief measures altogether. A devout Buddhist, for example, might observe that pain has something to teach us and to remove it entirely is unhelpful.

Reflection used to understand others, then, has to be of a more speculative kind and is needed to explore possibilities and ideas that arise out of a situation. The nurse examines their first premises about what the patient was feeling, attempting or dealing with and then rehearses other possibilities that present through reflecting on practice. This is a place where reflection becomes very clearly a part of critical thinking. The nurse reflects not only on that encountered, but also that which could apply there, as in the following example.

Case study: Carl's reflections on Martha's home care

Martha has been home from hospital now for several weeks. The ulcer on her leg is healing and her appetite seems to have improved. But she is struggling to interact with the home care workers who come in three times a day to assist with activities of daily living. The care workers report that she is withdrawn and they wonder whether she might be depressed, having dealt so long with the leg ulcer. As the visiting community nurse, Carl accepts that older patients in particular do sometimes suffer from depression, but he wonders too what the experience of care may have been like. He knows that a variety of carers have gone in to assist Martha and she has always been a very private sort of woman. What if she is struggling with care by strangers? It could be that she finds it rather hard to reveal her concerns to a succession of different people. Each of the care encounters is short, perhaps 15–20 minutes long.

continued ...

So building a rapport with carers could be very difficult. Carl reflects that sometimes care staff need quick cooperation. But this would be to meet staff needs. Simply assuming the patient has a problem, that she is depressed when she is not talkative, might be to jump to a conclusion. In deliberating on this Carl draws on his experience of other patients, but as well upon his own felt need sometimes to complete care in the most time-efficient way possible.

Understanding the profession or service

It may surprise you to discover that reflection has a part to play in understanding your chosen profession and service, and there will be opportunities within your course, through debates and seminars as well as through clinical practice, to reflect on what 'nursing is all about'. Such opportunities provide a chance to revisit how nursing seems to change. Part of what sustains you as a practitioner concerns clear ideas about what nurses do, what expertise they bring and what is different about the practice of the nurse. These are important considerations in a healthcare world where nurses are asked to diversify the sorts of work they engage in and where financial or other constraints might shape what the nurse can achieve (Allen, 2015).

Challenging assumptions

Reflection plays a major role in changing practice and changing profession over time. Healthcare work is not static, it evolves incrementally, and what was once seemingly ideal becomes suspect and anachronistic later. For example, if you were to read nursing textbooks from the 1960s, you would discover that nursing care was perceived as a supplemental activity to treatment and both were often prescribed by the medical consultant in charge. Today, nurses are much more strategic and engage in the design of health care, combining different sorts of knowledge (Christensen, 2011). We have greater autonomy, but also more responsibility.

One of the best uses of reflection is, then, at conference, at study day, or when reading a report or policy associated with nursing, to ascertain (a) whether this reflects your current understanding of best practice, and (b) whether, in the light of what you have encountered there, you need to change. Reflection in this context is often best conducted as part of a group of nurses, and especially where local protocols or best practice guidelines are formulated. Working in concert with others, you are more likely to formulate an informed opinion and to counterbalance the first negative emotional response that can arise when you are invited to change. As a student, you may have opportunities to join team meetings and discussion groups where just such reflections are under way.

Activity 2.4	Reflection

In a paper on the planning of future healthcare services, Carr et al. (2011) highlight the importance of experience, that which makes good sense of the client and practitioner requirements of a healthcare environment. Imagine that you are at a conference and about *continued ...* •••

> to challenge a speaker who advocates change on the basis of everything but experience. Jot down three arguments that you would make to argue in favour of experience based health-care design, that which might be discovered through reflection.

Some of our arguments were in areas such as client satisfaction, informed consent, avoidance of burnout among healthcare staff and balancing economic and quality care priorities. Reflection is key in each of these areas, understanding what sustains and develops services to coherent effect.

Making reflection work for you

Having defined reflection and made the case for its importance in nursing, we now consider how you can make reflection work for you. Table 2.1 sets out what we recommend at this stage. We then proceed to examine what is involved in association with each of our recommendations.

There are important points to make about Table 2.1. The first concerns wide-ranging reflection versus purposeful reflection. Some of the frameworks used by students to conduct and record their reflections focus tightly on the episode itself. You might accumulate a large number of unrelated reflective episode records. It is then more difficult to determine what the collection of reflective episodes add up to. A better strategy is to focus reflections on some important discourses

Recommendation	Notes
Clarify the purpose of your reflection on each occasion you use it.	However exciting it may seem to reflect freely and openly about events, in practice your thinking will be focused better if you have a stated purpose for the reflection. By asking a question, you will scrutinise events more closely, e.g. why was the patient so pleased with our care during her asthma crisis?
Reflect when you are most ready.	Reflection is often hard work and may provoke uncomfortable emotions. It is important to select the best times to reflect, when you feel emotionally calm, and where you have found the right space to conduct such work. Reflecting when you are still angry, for instance, will usually produce a record of what was wrong with the situation, rather than what you have learned yourself.
Identify confidantes with whom you are comfortable reflecting.	While it is possible to reflect on your own, it is also possible to delude yourself about a situation. It is better to reflect with a trusted colleague.
Allocate sufficient time and attention for the enterprise.	Reflection is a meditative activity requiring as much thinking time as writing time. It is wise to allocate at least 30–60 minutes to produce one or more thoughtful reflections – those that can prove useful later.

(Continued)

(Continued)

Recommendation	Notes
Use a reflective framework that works for you and is accepted by the university.	There are a wide variety of reflective frameworks and some university faculties direct what you should use. Try to work with one that helps you explore your experiences and thoughts in a way that makes sense to you. If it does not, you are less likely to engage in regular reflection.
Create reflective records you can use again.	To use reflective records later, you need to include enough contextual details to understand the events in question. Make sure you remind yourself what was happening, when the events occurred and what resources or support were available. Date the record to help you sense any changes in your perspective that occur over time.
In making and using such records, respect the rights of others.	In making reflective records, you necessarily refer to other people, so ensure you make anonymous their names and roles. It is important to store records securely and ensure you do not unfairly defame others.

Table 2.1: First principles of successful reflection

within nursing, those that help you to examine what might improve practice in the future. By exploring the accounts of patients, relatives and practitioners, those that set and implement policy, you will be better placed to examine what nurses can do to improve the quality of healthcare services (Hsu and McCormack, 2012). You will start to speculate cautiously about narratives and why problems exist and how opportunities have been or could be seized. A strategic use of reflection, for example on themed care encounters, is likely to offer greater rewards.

To help you to develop a strategic use of reflection, it is a good idea to begin with one or more questions to direct your attention. For example, 'What influences whether patients comply with my guidance on medication?' or 'What seems to increase patients' satisfaction with my explanations of treatment?' with regard to the theme of supporting grieving individuals that might be, 'What is my role in helping others manage their grief?' or 'How might I better assess a grieving person's needs?'

Activity 2.5   *Group working*

A useful way to share some reflection is to focus on an area with which most adult learners have some experience. Most people have some experience of grief (be it for a lost relative or friend; for changed circumstances, such as divorce; for the loss of a pet), so this can be a good starting point from which to explore some themed reflections within a group, in order to focus your thinking.

continued …

Start by all cataloguing individually your perceptions of what grief is and what is needed in terms of support. Writing points down will help to map the range of ways in which grief and support are understood.

Share your thoughts with the group. Do the points other people have raised expand your understanding?

Now go to: **www.helpguide.org/articles/grief-loss/coping-with-grief-and-loss.htm** and read the handout from the Helpguide organisation. See how they characterise grief and what seems helpful.

Compare notes: how well did your reflections on personal experience equip you to address what this organisation sees as important? What does the exercise teach you about the adequacy or otherwise of reflection without enquiry?

Students sometimes ask what is the right number of reflections to make and record within a given module or clinical placement. What is important is the quality of the reflections (something aided by linking each to a purpose) and their fit with the learning outcomes set. It is often better to prepare fewer but more fully developed reflections and those drawn from times when you feel fresh and inquisitive. So much the better if these cover a number of different purposes, helping you explore the diversity of nursing work.

While some deeply analytical individuals can and do conduct private reflections, the majority benefit from working with a chosen confidante. Clinical placements provide a mentor that you ought to consult, and students are allocated a personal tutor. A good confidante is someone who is willing to take an interest in your experience and learning and who has your trust, even though they sometimes challenge your thinking. Successful confidantes can usually be pictured responding to your reflection: 'yes … you could look at it that way and it has these merits. But have you also thought about …?' The confidante helps you see situations from different perspectives, and determine what you will observe and think about next.

As well as thinking about how much time you allocate for reflecting, consider too the sequence of thinking and writing. In part, you are thinking even as you write, but this has the disadvantage that, as your thoughts arrive on the page or screen, further thoughts, sometimes contradictory ones, are triggered. It could be this, it could be that. This was important, but then again perhaps it was not. Therefore it seems beneficial to allow yourself thinking-only time, or perhaps 'think and jot ideas down' time, so you can play with the possibilities before you. While the final written reflection does not necessarily need to be highly polished, it should be sufficiently accessible and coherent for you to use it to revise care later. For that reason, we advise thinking and drafting thoughts first, then penning refined reflective records. Both spontaneous notes and final reflections can be recorded in your portfolio (offering a full audit trail of thought).

Activity 2.6   *Research*

Investigate which reflective framework is recommended in association with your course. Discuss with your tutor what is expected in association with each of the headings there, and whether the course permits any latitude with regard to how you set out your records. Establish whether the framework recommended allows you to state clearly the purpose of your reflection, or whether you need to add this as a preliminary introduction.

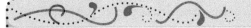

Chapter summary

This chapter has explored reflection as a form of critical thinking, one that focuses in particular upon experience and takes into account the emotions associated with experience, as well as an account of empirical events. Episodes of care are connected to the wider healthcare service and quality by the understanding of narratives and discourses.

In practice, reflection seems like two skills in one. If we reflect in action, we are thinking on our feet and reading practice situations as quickly and as accurately as possible. If we reflect on action, we use the benefits of hindsight but need to beware that reflecting too long after an event can result in problems associated with memory. By practising both skills, you will become better equipped to use experience to professional advantage, to understand how your perceptions relate to others, and to appreciate how this can then improve your understanding of your work as a nurse. While it is unrealistic to analyse all experiences in situ (you would suffer from information overload), it is possible to accumulate reflections after events, increasing your insights into your motives, actions and the consequences of what you do.

Reflection involves a process and several activities, for example deciding when to reflect, identifying a purpose, choosing how to frame the reflection and making a record. In support of that, we have shared a series of what we suggest are best principles associated with this work. It is important to work with university reflective frameworks, as reflection is itself a part of the curriculum and the ways in which students are expected to learn.

Further reading

Bassot, B (2013) *The Reflective Journal: Capturing your learning for personal and professional development.* Basingstoke: Palgrave Macmillan.

This accessible and empathetic book looks at the journaling element of reflection, but also offers a good summary of reflective practice and the different models of reflection you might be encouraged to use on your course.

Bolton, G (2014) *Reflective Practice: Writing and professional development,* 4th ed. Los Angeles, CA: Sage.

This book emphasises writing as an active reflective writing process, the very act of summarising events and perceptions being seen as professionally valuable. There is helpful material on learning journals and solutions to assessment problems.

Howatson-Jones, L (2016) *Reflective Practice in Nursing,* 3rd ed. London: Sage/Learning Matters.

This practical guide majors on the use of reflection in practice in a range of settings, the development of more inquisitive and speculative approaches to nursing care and ethical ways to make reflective practice records.

Useful websites

www.participatorymethods.org/method/reflective-practice

Participatory Methods is an organisation interested in many forms of social and economic development. We alert you to this website because reflective practice and action learning are means by which it is argued people from different backgrounds and with different expertise can collaborate to better the lot of others.

www.perceptionlab.com

The website of a group of St Andrews University researchers working in the field of human perception. Many of the papers and debates running on this site are associated with how we read other people. There is much to stimulate discussion about what you need to determine as part of the process of reflection.

Additional Online Material — For examples of analytical essays and other useful material, please visit the companion website at **www.sagepub.co.uk/price_harrington**

Chapter 3
Scholarly writing

NMC Standards for Pre-registration Nursing Education

This chapter addresses the following competencies.

Domain 2: Communication and interpersonal skills

3. All nurses must use the full range of communication methods, including verbal, non-verbal and written, to acquire, interpret and record their knowledge and understanding of people's needs. They must be aware of their own values and beliefs and the impact this may have on their communication with others. They must take account of the many different ways in which people communicate and how these may be influenced by ill health, disability and other factors, and be able to recognise and respond effectively when a person finds it hard to communicate.

7. All nurses must maintain accurate, clear and complete records, including the use of electronic formats, using appropriate and plain language.

Domain 4: Leadership, management and team working

2. All nurses must systematically evaluate care and ensure that they and others use the findings to help improve people's experience and care outcomes and to shape future services.

Chapter aims

After reading this chapter, you will be able to:

- summarise what we mean by scholarly writing relating this to different levels of learning;
- discuss the key features of essay structure and how these facilitate your explanation of learning achieved to date;
- explore the ways in which past experiences of writing can shape assumptions about academic writing in the future;
- make a clear case for 'thinking time' when preparing to write an academic paper;
- identify areas within your own writing where there is future scope for development.

Introduction

We start this chapter with three observations to reassure you. First, writing in a scholarly way seems to us a relatively new skill for most students. Thus, what we think of as the 'craftwork of writing' deserves help and support. Even though you may have written academic essays at school, it is less likely that these will also have been vocational works; that is, papers written about a practice such as nursing. Moreover, your past writing is likely to have operated at one level in the UK, that is at Advanced level in England, Wales or Northern Ireland or at Higher level in Scotland. Within an undergraduate pre-registration nursing degree, your thinking and writing will need to progress through different levels, higher education certificate, higher education diploma and first degree level. It is then reasonable to concede that scholarly writing, that which conveys critical thinking, deserves some thought and help from tutors and writers such as us. Second, writing in a scholarly way can be successfully learned provided that you take a little time to consider the process of work before you. While there are several different writing formats used within nursing courses (such as writing reflectively, writing about theory, writing plans and reports, evaluations of evidence), all are open to analysis, and students can and do improve their writing with practice. We return to different formats of writing in Part 3 of this book. Third, the writing skills you learn here will serve you well for the rest of your career. You will be surprised just how often they are used in the future, whether that is in association with courses of study, writing for publication or perhaps preparing reports associated with your work as a nurse.

Stewart, Fatima, Raymet and Gina (the students you met in Chapter 1) support the contentions shared here but, like other students, they sometimes find writing difficult. Stewart came to nursing from a career in commerce, where his writing was much more sparing and less reflective than is often required here. Fatima and Raymet note that they not only wrestle with writing in the required nursing form but also with some of the conventions of academic discussion as presented in British universities. There were different traditions of writing where they studied before, in India and Botswana, where their schooling focused on writing about factual knowledge and was less philosophical than is often required in nursing. Gina thinks that she begins with the clearest possible start point, as she is not used to any other tradition in writing. She has the most recent experience of secondary education, but she does not feel that this experience has equipped her for the higher level and applied nature of nursing programmes. She also feels that she lacks the life experience of the others to draw on in her writing, something often required in nursing. Their personal tutors have acknowledged the various challenges they all face, observing that students who move between one career, culture or educational system and another need help to adapt to the expectations of their new environment. Within a course of nursing studies, there may be many different forms of writing required – that which is reflective, analytical or strategic in nature. Irrespective of which background students come from, then, new skills will have to be learned and past assumptions about writing reconsidered. Conventions of reasoning and writing in the university where the student studies now, and those that guide judgements about good work there, need to be understood if students are to succeed.

In this chapter, we work with the experiences of Stewart and his colleagues, and lead you through different aspects of scholarly writing. This involves the connection of critical thinking and reflection to the conventions of scholarly discourse. We examine the ways in which you might best represent what you have reasoned and reflected upon. We begin this work with a brief but important introduction to different levels of learning and the taxonomies (classifications of learning level) that shape course design. It is important to understand that universities classify learning in different ways, so you will need to confer with your personal tutor to understand the course expectations in the different stages of your study. Sometimes the expectations of learning in the first, second and third or fourth year of a course are difficult to distinguish from one another. Confusingly, coursework assessments may, for example, use some descriptors such as 'critically discuss' across levels of learning, so it is hard to determine what the examiners expect. It is our recommendation that course leaders set out the learning taxonomies used in a course with students at the outset of their studies, so that students can better understand expectations as the course progresses. To help you with discussions with your course leader and personal tutor, however, we venture our own taxonomy of critical thinking and of reflection that relates specifically to applications of thinking discussed in Chapters 1 and 2. We use them here and in Part 3 of this book to better example how thinking might become more sophisticated as a course progresses.

The levels of learning matter set aside, we next examine how best to prepare for writing. We discuss the basic structure of academic pieces of work. While this will vary, dependent upon the format of writing that you are asked to engage in, we believe that there are some opening tenets of good writing that can be learned here. Lastly, we discuss what we mean by 'academic voice'. We use this term based on the research of the first of the authors of this book, where it was discovered that students need to understand the way in which they wish to present their learning to others (Price, 2003b). Sometimes we need to convey what others have discovered, and sometimes we need to convey our own philosophy, but most often we need to write to very disciplined purpose, demonstrating our command of the teaching provided. The clearer you are about academic voice, the better able you will be to link learning to written work.

Levels of learning

Whilst most students experience assessment work as a series of hurdles to be completed, universities structure work in a quite specific way. Less taxing assessments are designed to appear at the start of the course and more exacting ones towards the end. As the subject matter studied changes, this progression might not be quite so apparent to you. You may note easy and hard subjects and that might effectively cloak what the educators are working to achieve. In principle, though, less exacting ways of thinking and reflecting are tolerated at the start of your studies and then, when you have been taught more skills and have been practised in academic writing for longer, you are expected to demonstrate more sophisticated reasoning. Just what is expected across the university sector is quality assured by government agencies. In England, Wales and Northern Ireland, this is set out within the Further and Higher Qualifications Framework (Quality Assurance Agency for Higher Education, 2008) whereas in Scotland it is set out in the Framework for Qualifications in Higher Education Institutes In Scotland (Quality Assurance Agency Scotland, 2014). These frameworks characterise the learning achievements that might be expected at higher education certificate, diploma, first degree and master's degree levels.

The above frameworks cover a wide range of subjects across the university sector. Referring to these guidelines, faculties may then draw up taxonomies of learning that describe achievement at different levels specific to their subject areas. Some classic taxonomies have formed the basis of much academic thinking. In 1956, for example, Bloom devised a taxonomy for both cognitive (reasoning) and affective (that involving emotions) learning (Bloom et al., 1956), work that was adjusted more recently by Anderson and Krathwohl (2001). Our purpose here is not to share a history of learning taxonomies, but it is valuable to understand how they work, so Figure 3.1 shows a taxonomy used in the cognitive domain by Anderson and Krathwohl (2001).

What this diagram tells us is that it is considered much more sophisticated to understand than to remember something and that both are trumped by being able to apply your thinking to a context. That context might be clinical practice but it also might mean a new area of discourse, so, for example, the understanding of research shifts as we think of its different applications. Research designed to predict behaviour is different from research that explores how people make sense of their lives. The design of research differs according to context. Analysis is considered more sophisticated than applied reasoning and the ability to evaluate and create trumps all other reasoning that might be expected of the student. The assessments that you complete will operate at one or other level within a taxonomy such as this and that level can typically be spotted by words used in the assignment question. So, for example, if you are asked to simply list and define something, your learning is being assessed at the remembering or understanding level. If you are asked to interpret something, to apply it to a practice context, your reasoning is being assessed at the application level. If you are asked to appraise or debate a subject, then you are being asked to analyse. If you are asked to design something, then you are invited to reason at the creative level. The often used 'critically discuss' assignment instruction can be confusing because, in this taxonomy, *discuss* is usually associated with comprehension and understanding and *critically* is associated with analysis or evaluation. We make the point to emphasise the importance of discussing assessment question requirements with module leaders and personal tutors.

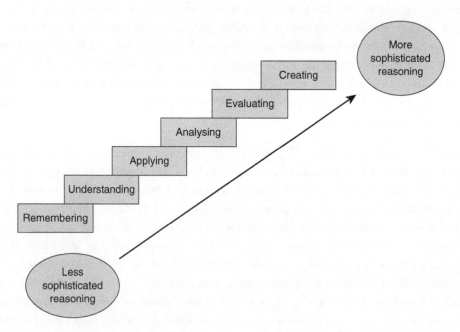

Figure 3.1: Cognitive learning taxonomy (based on the findings of Anderson and Krathwohl, 2001)

Activity 3.1   *Reflection*

Look back in your course handbook to see what learning outcomes have been set for your course and how these change as you progress from year one to year two and so on through the modular programme of studies. Do the learning outcomes associated with the later modules of your study seem harder? Is there a greater emphasis on creativity and the ability to evaluate? Are you meant to deal with more ambiguous information in the later stages of your course?

Reader feedback on the previous edition of this textbook suggests that it might help students to see taxonomies of critical thinking and of reflection, which better help them to distinguish between different levels of achievement. Remember, these exist to facilitate your discussions with your tutors, to clarify what counts as more sophisticated reasoning and reflection. They need to always be studied in conjunction with course learning outcomes and individual assessment requirements. With such caveats noted, we have ventured two taxonomies below.

We have been persuaded by Baxter-Magolda's (1992) explanation of levels of reasoning, which captures what some of you may have already encountered in Benner's (2001) account of the growth of nurses as reflective and intuitive individuals. In the least sophisticated forms of reasoning, individuals are inflexible and rule-governed, seeing only one explanation, one point of view. As reasoning becomes more sophisticated it becomes first transitional (other possibilities are accommodated) and then contextual. The reasoning is nuanced, and it relates to a given set of circumstances. It is not that theories are not valuable, it is that they need to be understood in the context of need or use. Fink (2009), in his description of learning, emphasises just how important 'situational factors' are. Much of what we must understand and do is negotiated in context. There is often no absolute right answer in health care, only safer conclusions and more appropriate ways forward. At the pinnacle of reasoning is independent thought. For our purposes, we can think of independent thinking as that which has a vision for better practice, which shows the nurse 'thinking outside the box' and with due regard for patient safety. Independent thought reframes information in ways that enable the nurse to see problems or challenges afresh and to identify new opportunities.

We can link the Baxter-Magolda (1992) levels of reasoning to the applications of critical thinking and reflecting discussed in Chapters 1 and 2 of this book. We have combined the two into two tables, one for critical thinking and one for reflection in Tables 3.1 and 3.2. In studying these tables, we think that you should anticipate that the highest order critical thinking and reflections skills will develop in full during the later modules of your study. Contextual thinking, for example, cannot be anticipated until you have had chance to apply concepts and ideas, either in practice or perhaps in case studies, debates and action-learning sessions completed in class. Independent thinking is often associated with project work, something that is classically used to complete a level of study or your degree as a whole. Less sophisticated reasoning is never sought but is more likely to be accommodated in the earlier modules of study. Tutors and assessors are not naive; they understand that until your reasoning has been facilitated through debates and discussions, through seminars and tutorials, it is unrealistic to expect advanced reasoning. While this all might seem a little daunting, remember that we learn to reason better as part of a well-designed course. You are not expected to be an independent thinker from the outset. We return once again to these tables in Part 3 of this book, as we discuss the ways to demonstrate more sophisticated reasoning in your written coursework.

Activity 3.2   *Critical thinking*

Study Tables 3.1 and 3.2. What do you think it will feel like to progress upwards through these levels of critical thinking and reflection? Make a note of any concerns you might have and wish to raise with your personal tutor. If you already think you have progressed beyond 'absolute reasoning' in several areas, excellent! But what enables you to reach that conclusion? What can you point to as evidence? In our experience, many students move upwards into transitional thinking quite quickly in their course of studies, but some elements of reasoning can and do stubbornly refuse to develop. Personal tutors want to work with you to understand where and how well you progress.

Preparing to write

Having elucidated different levels of reasoning and reflecting, we now turn to the business of preparing to write. Every time you prepare a piece of coursework you are selecting information to share, ways of expressing yourself which demonstrate that you have met the module learning outcomes and have made progress in your reasoning and reflection. Students are surprised by the emphasis we place upon preparation time, imagining that we compose as we write. In our experience, there is real benefit in allocating 'thinking time' before you write. This is not simply a matter of making a plan, it is about distilling your thoughts before you try to use them to represent your learning. Tutors regularly comment that they can see in academic essays where students are thinking as they write. Problems include the following.

- Not answering the question set, or preparing the wrong sort of coursework.

- Allocating the word count poorly within the essay (early sections getting the lion's share of attention and later sections suffering).

- Material being presented in an incompletely reasoned state (it is hard to go back and edit an essay when you fear that, in doing so, you may lose the plot and write something inferior).

- Essay conclusions falling short of requirements because students have argued many things but have never quite determined what they think.

- Using others' work and representing it as your own (plagiarism is much more likely where you have allocated insufficient time to the preparation of work. It is tempting to 'borrow' the words of others, failing to acknowledge the source or at least to use quotation marks ('') when you present the exact words of another author).

	Absolute thinking	Transitional thinking	Contextual thinking	Independent thinking
Asking questions	Few or no questions asked, information accepted as fact.	Questions asked about whether claims are correct, whether other possibilities might exist.	Nuanced questions asked, those applying to a circumstance or need. Typically, these relate to a patient, a plan or practice and its protocols.	Imaginative new questions are asked, those that reframe the topic, problem or issue in some way, liberating nurses to suggest fresh ideas.
Discriminating	There is little or no discrimination about what is right, best or proven. The student simply rehearses what others have taught.	Knowledge is seen as contentious in some regard; there are other possibilities to debate. The student writes about why something may be preferred, understanding the interplay of premises, conclusions and evidence, how these can help determine whether arguments are supportable.	Information is interrogated with regard to its fit within a circumstance or need. Theories are applied, concepts examined and combined with experience to explore what works.	Judgements on best information to use are now refined, articulating a range of influencing factors the student is taking into account. The student takes an overview of issues in the round.

Interpreting and speculating	At best the student selects elements of information to include in their report of what is right, best, common sense. Interpretation rarely extends to why some information is more relevant than others. Speculation is rarely seen at this level as the thinking is rule governed.	Speculation is apparent as the student considers different arguments about what is important, what is happening or needed. The written account clearly exhibits discussion of why one option is better than another. The nurse demonstrates the need to interrogate theory rather than accept it pat.	Interpretation involves the mixing of multiple sources of information, theory, research, experience and protocol. The review of information is conducted with regard to a clear purpose or goal. Speculations centre on what information can or should be used, what is needed in the context explored.	Independent thinking involves admission of information or ideas to a discussion that are entirely relevant, but which most would not have considered. The thinker questions what is given, what is a problem or need and what might represent a solution or opportunity. The nurse speculates about what could be possible with reference to the highest standards of professional practice.
Making arguments	The arguments of others are put forward and without question.	An array of arguments are presented, showing awareness of options. The merits of different arguments are outlined. The nurse determines which of the competing arguments is most credible.	The nurse's own arguments are advanced and with context, examining what is needed, ethical, relevant, realisable and coherent as information is reviewed. Arguments may be combined from different places in order to build a convincing case for what can, might or should be done now.	Strikingly new arguments are presented, showing how the nurse has conceived of information in a fresh new way. Arguments are cogent, coherently and compellingly rehearsed so the reader feels they have learned something important and even liberating.

Table 3.1: A taxonomy of critical thinking

	Absolute thinking	Transitional thinking	Contextual thinking	Independent thinking
Celebrating practice	The reasoning is trite, there is only one version of best practice and why that has merit is not discussed.	Success is seen like the curate's egg, it was good in part. Focus shifts to what worked and why, but it is acknowledged that not all practice was perfect.	The nurse examines why practice succeeded and with reference to the experience of different stakeholders.	The very way in which practice is conceived, what the nurse and others are trying to do is engaged in the discussion of success. Practice is understood in terms of values, that which seems quintessential and of the highest quality.
Correcting practice	Practice problems are not acknowledged or if they are they are ascribed to the behaviour of others alone. There is no ownership of issues that need attention.	Shortfalls and problems that lead to the substandard practice are articulated, including those of the nurse themselves. The reflection impresses as inquisitive, honest and it articulates why elements of practice are problematic.	The reflection on shortfalls and problems is nuanced, and relates directly to the issues that are of most concern in a given practice context. The work demonstrates how the nurses think about what others hoped for and sets this against what they were trying to achieve.	Correcting practice involves a critical examination of beliefs, values and attitudes, the assumptions and ideology that might shape care delivery. Independent thinkers are brave enough to explore these more fundamental issues as part of a practice review.
Understanding self	There is little or no introspection, behaviour is often thought of as common sense.	The nurse explores questions about why they thought or acted as they did, and the way this affects their approach to care.	The reasonableness of the nurse's approach in a given context is now honestly addressed. The nurse recognises that she has to be metacognitive, that is to understand how she negotiates care, and how that might or might not be suitable to changing circumstances of health care.	Experience is understood as an opportunity to re-examine the nurse's own values, beliefs and attitudes. The account shows the nurse questioning that in her or himself that affects their expertise, their readiness or their fit to particular elements of practice.

Understanding others	Others are understood in stereotypical terms and usually with reference to roles. Patients are like this, doctors are like that.	Others are understood in the round, as individuals, and usually with a history, background or training, that helps to shape how they see practice. Individuals are respected for what they experience, do or achieve.	Others are understood as actors in a situation, those that must make sense of encounters that they have and who have emotions, beliefs and values of their own that influence how they read care encounters. The account is insightful and empathetic.	Others are perceived as individuals making sense of their existence, with their own philosophy and culture or traditions. The rightness of care, the best fit of support is understood in terms of helping the patient, relative or professional colleague in their own journey.
Understanding profession and service	Service and profession are understood in stereotypical terms and usually without obvious insight into how the nurse's own opinion might affect reputation. The nurse might 'label' what others do.	Profession and service are understood as complex and involving a lot of different contributions. Consideration shifts as to why the profession or service is as it is, how and why it may be shifting.	Professions and service are understood as in transit, working with a society and with patients whose needs are also changing. The fit might not be perfect, tensions are articulated and the nurse exhibits a shared responsibility in improving performance.	Healthcare service is understood as a culturally mediated and negotiated process. Standards of practice as articulated by governing bodies have to be understood, and interpreted soundly in the face of changing healthcare demands. There is an imaginative and a committed engagement in best standards of care.

Table 3.2: A taxonomy of reflection

Activity 3.3   *Critical thinking*

We asked our students to each consider one of the preparations in Figure 3.2 that we think of as important in scholarly writing. Your challenge is to identify the opportunities you have to engage in such preparatory work. Where do your opportunities exist to think about an academic essay in preparation?

Coming from a different professional background, Stewart is already attuned to the need to understand the writing task set. Nursing courses include a wide variety of forms of writing and each is closely associated with reasoning in different ways. For example, if you are asked to present a portfolio of learning, you will need to write reflectively but you will also need to include elements of strategy as you present plans for developing your work in the future. We suggest not only that you read the requirements carefully (the assignment brief, the report required by a manager, etc.) but also that you take time to clarify any concerns and queries with the person who set the brief. Pay particular attention to the wording of assessment questions. Does the assignment brief what is really required by 'critically discuss' for instance? If you fail to clarify such matters and guess the requirements, mistakes can prove costly in terms of grades achieved.

Many of you may empathise with Fatima's response about the difficulty of adopting a position within a piece of coursework. In the past, students have often been required to summarise what others have said, especially teachers. Looking back to Table 3.1 and its points on making arguments, you can see that this represents absolutist thinking and something more is typically required in an undergraduate module. Past courses may have been more pedagogical, assigning the teacher a greater role, confirming either what can fairly be supported or what is most acceptable. In yet other courses, teachers have more of a facilitation role, and are charged with prompting the students to work through issues to reach their own conclusions. The move from a background where teaching was more prominent, to one where the facilitation of learning predominates, is difficult for students (Cortazzi and Jinn, 1997). In our experience, this is heightened in many areas of the nursing curriculum, where students are required to 'adopt a position', to 'take a stance on an issue' of their own. For example, in rehabilitation, where work is shared with patients and lay carers, you might be asked to state what represents a reasonable level of support. What do you expect patients or relatives to learn and do, and what do you think we as nurses should contribute? In these and similar matters, you do need to make a case and it is then important for you to be completely clear about this before you start. It takes time to discover and settle on your position before writing.

In Figure 3.2, Raymet's points are important: students often wonder when an argument becomes a fact. Moreover, if you are to grapple with a series of arguments, how should they best be arranged?

In nursing courses, it is often necessary to present a series of arguments, each of which supports the case or position we adopt. You will often find within UK universities that the case or position is stated early within the academic paper and the main text then used to rehearse arguments and counter arguments, which help the student to sum up insights within their conclusion (there are other approaches within reflective writing; we explore these approaches elsewhere).

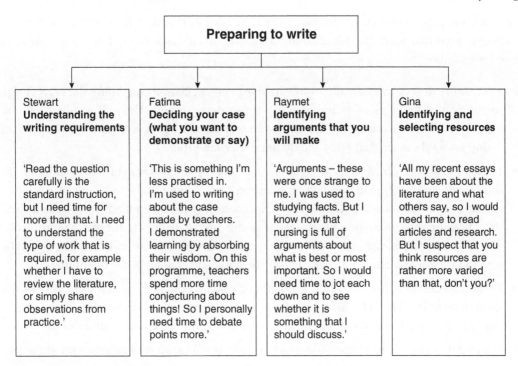

Figure 3.2: Preparing to write

Such essays are typical of what tests transitional or contextual thinking (see Table 3.1). For example, your case or position may be that nurses should educate patients to take on self-care activities. Arguments in support of this then include: (a) that patients gain independence through their own learning; (b) that it is not economically viable to go on delivering all the care, so patients and relatives need to develop their own skills; and (c) that patients develop greater self-esteem through the process of learning to care for themselves. This may or may not be your experience of previous learning, where perhaps you revealed your position incrementally at the end of your paper. However, the case-first sequence is the reasoning norm for more philosophical essays within nursing, so if you have difficulties making that transition, it is worth discussing the adjustments you are trying to make with your personal tutor.

Gina is correct that we envisage students using a variety of resources as part of their academic writing and that it takes time to select what will be included in a piece of coursework. Observations from practice, arguments articulated by others in interview, and hospital care philosophies are just a few of the things that could support what you write about. It takes time to evaluate each of these and to judge how each resource will be linked to the arguments made (*this* supports my argument, *that* reminds us there are alternative perspectives).

Avoiding plagiarism

Plagiarism is the use of other people's written work, figures, tables or diagrams, and the representation of these as your own work within an academic paper. Plagiarism carries severe penalties at university. At the least, you may receive a written warning; at worst, you may have an academic paper failed or be dismissed from the course. It is therefore vital to prepare for writing in ways that limit the risk of committing plagiarism. Each of the following represents good preparation.

- Find and read very carefully the university rules and regulations regarding the correct representation of the work of others within your academic essays. This will usually be found within your course handbook or the study skills section of the course website. Make a point of asking tutors about anything that you do not understand there.

- Use a notebook to record all the sources of information you have used, including websites. Do this immediately when you find helpful material. Make a note of the web address (its URL) so that you can find it again. One of the temptations is to use notes made from websites and then, because you cannot find the reference details later, to represent the words used as your own. If you find a passage of text that seems helpful, then photocopy or print the page and be sure to write the reference for the article or the book and chapter at the top of that.

- Do not assume that, because there is no author's name evident on a web page, it does not need to be referenced. The default position should be that where author details seem to be missing you should treat the organisation that runs the web page as the author of the work.

- Get into the habit of using quotation marks regularly ('') at the start and the end of the passage of copied words. If you paraphrase work (that is, rephrase the points in your own words), make sure that you do a thorough job. Changing just the odd word within the sentence does not constitute paraphrasing and you may be told that you have plagiarised work. Imagine that the original text that you read said this: 'Rehabilitation is both an educational and a support process, one in which the patient is required to actively engage and one which requires the nurse to strategise, evaluating how well the patient is doing and adjusting care accordingly.' You might paraphrase this as: 'nurses work strategically with patients, teaching and supporting them, adjusting rehabilitation work as they go.' The paraphrase captures the essence of what has been written without using the same words. You still then need to acknowledge the source, indicating the author's name and year of publication within brackets within the text.

- Reserve enough thinking time before you write. However daunting it seems, you do have to decide what *you* think about others' reported work. Examiners respect that your points will not always seem profound, but they do need to understand what sense you make of that which has been reviewed.

- Do not share essay drafts or past assignment answers with other students. There is a risk that others may copy your work and you could be charged with aiding and abetting them (academic collusion). Universities use software systems that can show the similarities between student work received, including that which was submitted in the past.

- Do not be tempted to purchase essay work from the internet – not only is this considered a calculated effort to cheat (one mandating a severe penalty) but also you may use something that is in any case not fit for purpose. Tutors are keenly aware of what you have written in the past, and what *this* essay requires, so subterfuge essays are often spotted.

- Check to see whether your university offers you access to a software script-checking service such as Turnitin (**http://turnitin.com**). Turnitin compares passages of your own work against that which exists within other published and website work, showing you where your words match those elsewhere. There is no problem with found matches where you have attributed the source of the material and used quotation marks appropriately, but where sentences or longer passages of your work match those from elsewhere and no attribution is recorded, vital corrections need to be made.

The basics of structure

Pieces of academic work have a beginning, a middle and an end, and must seem complete and coherent. It is this quality of completeness and coherence, together with authority, clarity and precision, that we search for when planning a paper. Completeness and coherence are supported by the way in which we structure the coursework, authority is determined by how we present and support arguments, and clarity and precision are affected by how we help others to navigate the paper, and through the way in which we decide what to include and what to leave out. Force too much information into an essay and clarity suffers.

Activity 3.4   *Research*

To help you to explore structure more fully, we have included an analytical essay within the Learning Matters website (**www.sagepub.co.uk/price_harrington**). Studying this essay will help you to examine the points we make below. If you do not have access to the web, you may prefer instead to examine an article published within a nursing journal. If you choose this second option, we recommend that you select an article that explores a topic (e.g., rehabilitation nursing), rather than one that reports research. While published works are more polished than those submitted for coursework assessment, they nevertheless include relevant structural features that we can discuss.

When you have selected a resource, refer to it and answer our questions at the end of each of the following sections.

Introducing the work

All pieces of academic work need an introduction, which has four roles:

- to identify the subject matter of the piece written;

- to secure the reader's attention and interest;

- to establish the writer's position or perspective;

- to set any contexts within which the paper needs to be understood.

It is possible to establish the subject matter by stating the essay question set or to simply say at the outset, 'This essay is written about the rehabilitation work of the nurse'. However, there are slightly more adventurous ways of introducing a subject. An academic essay is not journalism but, like journalists, we are required to interest our readers in the essay subject matter, even if they are examiners and are paid to read our work. We need a 'hook' to encourage them to read on.

Two common ways of doing this are:

- to start with a bold point that highlights the importance of the subject matter; for example: 'There is at least anecdotal evidence that nurses and patients are not always working to the same ends, regarding rehabilitation';

or

- to introduce a dilemma that needs to be addressed; for example: 'There is a problem with patient rehabilitation and this is linked to what we consider ideal and what seems possible given resource constraints'.

You will need to decide whether your introduction will be presented in the first person singular (referring to 'I') or in the third person, referring to 'the nurse' or 'nurses'. First person singular is the norm where any form of reflective writing is required. Where in the third person you refer to 'the author', it is important to beware of literature review traps. Are you talking about the author of other papers reviewed or to you, the author of this essay?

If your work concerns practice or an area of professional discourse (e.g., applied science or pharmacology), your introduction needs to make this clear. You might, for instance, refer to a client group your work concerns (such as postoperative patients) or a particular area of practice (e.g., the use of analgesia).

Activity 3.5   *Reflection*

Examine your chosen essay or article, to establish whether the introduction achieves all of the aims of an introduction, as listed above. If any of the key features are missing, what are the implications for the rest of the piece? Look back to Table 3.1 to examine what the introduction offers as regards levels of critical thinking. Can you see how setting out a case early on, focusing the essay, might help you to demonstrate clear arguments and to show how you are interpreting a subject?

Signposting the work

Towards the end of the introduction to your work, you need to help the reader to understand how the rest of the work is set out ('This essay is set out in the following sections …'). Signposting is not only a description of the rest of the work, though; it frequently includes an indication of the stance that you take and the purpose of your paper. You may indicate that this paper on rehabilitation nursing considers the role of the nurse in section 1 and the role of patients and lay carers in section 2, and then debates the liaison work between the two groups in section 3 ('The paper makes the case that rehabilitation is a negotiated activity and one that requires careful liaison between stakeholders').

Activity 3.6   *Critical thinking*

Did you spot signposting in the work that you chose to read? It frequently consists of just one very important paragraph at the end of the introduction. Does the signposting within your reviewed work help you to read forward with a clear purpose, knowing what the author is trying to do?

Developing the main body of the work

Classically, academic essays include a main text with few subsections, which rarely includes figures or tables. Within nursing, however, the conventions are rapidly changing and it is usual to arrange the work using subheadings to help the reader to navigate your work, and both figures and tables where these help you to make a point quickly and clearly. Check your course handbook to establish what are the local norms. Our own preference is to encourage writing that helps the reader to follow your arguments, and includes features that are similar to those used when writing for publication (section headings and tables or figures).

What remains important in academic papers is that you write in disciplined paragraphs, with short sentences that enable you to make clear points. Where you do use figures, tables or appendices, they must all be clearly referred to in the text and within brackets (e.g., 'see Figure 1', 'Table 3 refers', 'see Appendix 1').

What do we mean by a disciplined paragraph? In practical terms, it is one that:

- attends to a single subject (e.g., ascertaining the patient's readiness to rehabilitate);

- includes clear points, your own or others' arguments (e.g., 'While economic pressures exist to speed up rehabilitation, the readiness of a patient to learn skills still affects the pace of their progress');

- provides support for what has been stated. This is often where references to the literature come in but, as we have noted, other evidence gleaned from practice could be referred to (e.g., 'An example patient helps to make the case. Mr X reported that he felt paralysed by fear regarding taking exercise after his heart attack. He worried that staff had not completely understood the risks').

Sentences that extend beyond a couple of lines of text are much more likely to seem ambiguous to the reader. Being scholarly does not necessarily mean writing longer sentences or cramming more information into a paragraph.

The last key consideration regarding the main text is that you build a series of arguments. To demonstrate that you are thinking critically, it is important not to accept points at face value. For this reason, a paragraph that makes one argument could, in some instances, be followed by another paragraph that makes a second argument. But it is important by the end of your work to demonstrate that you have reached your own conclusions, even if this is only to suggest that the debate continues. Remember, in transitional and contextual reasoning, you will have to demonstrate possible arguments and to review their merits. You will need to determine the best-fit arguments to a context of interest, whether that be clinical practice or perhaps a review of nursing theories and their ease of use. So, turning once more to our example, we might spend one paragraph arguing the above point about the importance of patients' readiness to commence rehabilitation, and then add a second that reminds the reader that prolonged inactivity increases the risk of post-myocardial infarction complications. On balance, then, the recommended way forward is physical rehabilitation and consistent psychological support while patients test their limits.

Activity 3.7   *Critical thinking*

Examine your chosen essay or article, to identify some examples of what you think are especially successful paragraphs and to list the arguments you can see being developed within the main text of the paper. How does this structure compare with some of your own past essays? Can you see how the work starts to have a bigger impact on you because of its structure?

Reaching a conclusion

Academic coursework (unless otherwise instructed) requires a conclusion. Within the conclusion there should be no substantial new material. Its purpose is to sum up what has been written so far. However, the essay has to show what sense has been made about the arguments presented. Beyond all those points about helping the patient rehabilitate, what does this amount to? The author needs to deduce what the arguments support. Perhaps it is first to support patients, because they are doing a lot of the rehabilitation work. Perhaps it is to coordinate rehabilitation work. Perhaps it is that if physiotherapy is given before patient education has been delivered patient anxiety might be increased.

Activity 3.8   *Critical thinking*

Scrutinise your chosen paper to see whether the conclusion achieves the above. Do not be surprised if you identify some shortfalls here. Even published papers sometimes include weak conclusions. Did the conclusion make reference to a case that was stated at the start of the essay or article?

Adopting the right voice

We come at last to the business of 'voice'. You might be surprised that we use a term more associated with singing to describe scholarly writing. By *voice* we mean conveying your thoughts in such a way that your thinking is demonstrated as something that seems orderly, measured, critical or reflective, as the need dictates. Academic voice helps you to portray that you are thinking at a higher level of critical thinking. Singers use a voice to convey emotions or drama. Students need, through their texts, to use a voice to illustrate or represent their learning. We have already conveyed two ways in which your work will seem more scholarly – the first, developing a coherent structure for your work, and the second, building a series of arguments that demonstrate your reasoning. There remain, though, some important niceties in the ways in which you write (use your voice) that will enhance your reputation as a scholar.

Activity 3.9   *Critical thinking*

Look at some sample sentences that our four students used in their earliest essays. They are at pains to remind us that their work has improved since! There are some classic faults within these short extracts that demonstrate less than scholarly work, and we invite you to identify them.

Gina: *That patients wait, lying on trolleys within a corridor or a corner of casualty, is utterly appalling.*

Stewart: *Time is money, so the doctor's stay at the bedside is always short and patients ask others what has then been decided as regards their treatment.*

Raymet: *The assessment I made of the patient was holistic. I examined their rash and listened carefully to their anxieties.*

Fatima: *A tutor has explained that patients sometimes only want to please the nurse, rather than state their real concerns. This seems right to me.*

Did you spot the fact that, in Activity 3.9, Gina was using hyperbole; that is, accentuating a point made in a heavy-handed or excessive way. While we might share dismay at the length of time patients wait to secure a bed, and would not commend long waiting times and uncomfortable conditions, the conventions of academic writing are that we express opinion in rather more measured terms. In this example, a more measured critique of this situation might be to observe that the lengthy waits were undignified, that they brought into question the adequacy of resources, and that they raised questions about service standards. The phrase 'utterly appalling' appeals to the emotions of the reader rather than their intellect, and we do not convey analysis so clearly. A scholarly voice is measured – one where the writer does not move easily and quickly to emotional condemnation or superlatives ('the care was fantastic'), for example, when praising practice in another.

Stewart's fault in this example concerned what we call a colloquialism – that is, a form of short-hand writing that we assume the reader understands. 'Time is money' is a well-known aphorism that describes how people prioritise their time using economic considerations. But used in this context it hardly does justice to the doctor. There is certainly a problem here, because patients may need lengthy explanations of planned treatment, but this is a problem of time and resources, and says something too about information sharing and informed consent. 'Time is money' does not do justice to the matter and conveys (the unintended) message that some matters are obvious and can quickly be dismissed in an academic essay. Colloquial language often conveys the sort of absolutist thinking that are seen in Tables 3.1 and 3.2.

The fault in Raymet's writing is rather more subtle, but nonetheless a good example of where the scholarly voice has not yet been developed. If work is to be precise, it is necessary to use terms and concepts with care. In this instance, Raymet is referring to holism and claiming that the assessment of a patient was holistic. However, holistic refers to four major aspects of a person's life and experience: the physical, the psychological, the social and the spiritual. It suggests that the care delivered engages deeply and comprehensively with the patient's experience (Hudson, 2015). What Raymet reports here is not a holistic assessment of the patient but one that concentrates upon the rash (physical) and patient anxieties (psychological). No mention is made of spiritual concerns or social needs. It is important, then, to use terms precisely. Checking a dictionary can help to resolve this issue.

There are two possible problems with the academic voice in Fatima's extract. First, there are usually conventions associated with the referencing of sources and, here, Fatima is not following them. If she has been encouraged to include personal discourses with a tutor within academic work, it is necessary to state in brackets the nature of that (e.g., 'personal email communication with tutor X'). Second, students sometimes present work that is designed to please a tutor or other marker of the finished work. They may refer with approval to what the examiner has taught, said or written elsewhere. In scholarly writing, though, examiners wish to learn what the student has reasoned rather than what the tutor has taught. It is necessary to demonstrate your own judgement and evaluation of issues, rather than to simply approve those that you think might please someone else.

Thus, a scholarly voice is one that:

- acknowledges the source of points and perspectives of others (in the literature or elsewhere);
- demonstrates your own reasoning and reflection;
- uses terms precisely and consistently;
- expresses points in a measured rather than an emotive way;
- avoids forms of shorthand reasoning such as colloquialisms.

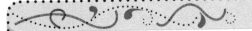

Chapter summary

We return to the matter of scholarly writing again in Part 3 of this book. It is important here, however, to acknowledge the above precepts of good writing, some of which can seem implicit rather than explained within the course that you study. Pausing to consider what is required of you by your tutor and the university, and where that fits and does not fit with what you have learned before, can help you to understand what seems more challenging about study. Most of what is required is determined by the need to convey your learning in as clear and accessible a manner as possible: by adhering to simple practices, by writing a paper that has a clear beginning, middle and end, and by using devices to guide the reader through the work. It is about considering how much information you can or should include within a sentence or paragraph, and whether your work within that paragraph has strayed away from its subject. It is certainly about good spelling and grammar, as well as checking work before it is submitted.

Of all the fundamental errors in scholarship writing that we see within nurse education programmes, there are three that recur frequently. Some students fail to appreciate what sort of writing they are asked to provide. Like Stewart, they need to clarify the requirements

continued ...

set, usually by taking questions to the tutor. Other students begin to write long before they have concluded what they think. Tables 3.1 and 3.2 emphasise just how important and complex thinking can be. Students are then hard pressed to identify what case they wish to present. 'Thinking time' is more important than 'writing time' and it is worth investing in, especially if you jot down notes about your developing ideas. A third group of students rush forward with their writing, failing to attend to the academic voice required within assignments. They use imprecise colloquial terms. The net effect is that their work seems ill considered and hurriedly prepared.

Many of the papers that students have criticised as 'too descriptive' are associated with such faults. Arguments are lacking and the ideas discussed have been handled in a shorthand way.

Examining examples of scholarly writing in different places will help you to identify what conveys learning clearly and well. By studying the resources associated with this chapter, or those that you find within the university library, you will be much better placed to represent your reasoning and reflection when it comes to work that carries course marks.

Further reading

By definition, we see a need for a book on reasoning, reflecting and writing in nursing (this one). There are, however, some other texts that we admire on the more general principles of essay writing. You would do well to look at these, if you wish to augment your reading of our chapters.

Greetham, B (2013) *How to Write Better Essays*, 3rd ed. Basingstoke: Palgrave Macmillan.

An accessible and logical guide to the business of finding information, making coherent notes and turning these into coherent and adequately source cited essays.

MacKevic, V (2012) *From Confusion to Conclusion: How to write a first class essay.* CreateSpace Independent Publishing Platform.

A refreshingly frank and considered guide that takes the reader back through what it takes to distil information found into text presented at the end. The book attends at some length to essays that examine research evidence, something of great importance in nursing.

McMillan, K and Weyers, J (2013) *How to Cite, Reference and Avoid Plagiarism at University.* Harlow: Pearson.

Universities provide guides on how to avoid plagiarism, but a fuller textbook is also useful. These authors show what the common mistakes are and highlight what is important in referencing websites (something it is easy to become confused about).

Useful websites

Each university produces its own guide to good academic writing process and sets out requirements for the way in which assignments should be presented. Conventions may differ by university. We therefore direct you to the study skills section of your university, rather than prompt you to a wider trawl of the internet.

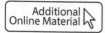

Additional Online Material

For examples of analytical essays and other useful material, please visit the companion website at **www.sagepub.co.uk/price_harrington**

Part 2
Critical thinking and reflecting in nursing contexts

Chapter 4
Making sense of lectures

....
∴ ⌒⌒ ∴   **NMC Standards for Pre-registration Nursing Education**

Because the subject matter of lectures varies widely, there are no specific standards to link
to. The skills covered in this chapter underpin how you successfully learn and achieve all
the standards, within the environment of lectures.
....

Chapter aims

After reading this chapter, you will be able to:

- detail ways to engage in the lecture so as to enhance the quality of your learning;
- summarise ways in which to prepare for a lecture;
- discuss the different ways of thinking in a lecture that might enrich your experience;
- explain why questions are so important to learning in a lecture;
- summarise important things to do after the lecture has ended.

Introduction

Nursing courses provide a range of learning opportunities, each of which enables you to discuss
ideas with others and explore issues that may have arisen through what you see and hear. Among
those learning opportunities, lectures make a major contribution. Lectures are well suited to
conveying significant amounts of information to large numbers of students and can, in skilful
hands, convey a great deal about how the nurse reasons (Quinn and Hughes, 2013). Lectures
are delivered in subject areas such as anatomy and physiology, pharmacology, nursing theory,
healthcare ethics and nursing management. Accomplished lecturers admit you into their own
thought processes and help you to explore the possibilities that they consider. You gain insight
into how a tutor weighs the pros and cons of issues, and determines what is of higher priority or
most significant in caring for patients. Because, in most instances, tutors talk more than students
within the lecture, there is a risk that your approach to learning could be unduly passive. It is
possible, for instance, to attend a lecture and to gain comparatively little from it, not necessarily
because the lecture was poorly delivered but because you did not focus inquisitively enough on
what was shared.

It is crucial that you gain the most from those lectures that you attend, especially where the
subject is not repeated later and subsequent teaching assumes that a subject has been grasped.

If you miss such opportunities, your future learning may be impaired and you might fail related assessments. The better organised you are as regards learning in lectures, the more you will derive from them.

In this chapter, we assist you to plan for forthcoming lectures and to arrive at each in an inquisitive state of mind. We describe the features of typical lectures and identify how best to arrive at a balance between listening, thinking, writing and communicating. In particular, we attend to learning associated with questions in the lecture – those that the tutor might pose to you and those that, in turn, you might want to ask. We finish the chapter with some work that you should undertake after the lecture has ended.

Activity 4.1   *Reflection*

No one supposes that every lecture is perfect. However, to help you to orientate discussions within this chapter, begin now by recalling a particularly successful lecture that you enjoyed. Identify what seemed to make the lecture such a success. Was success determined largely by the skills of the tutor, the contributions of the students, or a mixture of the two? What do you deduce from your part in that; what is it important for *you* to contribute?

Preparing for the lecture

Every lecture that you attend has the potential to enhance your thinking and to develop further your confidence as a nurse. However, it is not necessarily the case that you will let it. There are all sorts of potential barriers to successful learning in lectures and some of them are associated with our assumptions and expectations (Hudson, 2014). We may come to the lecture anxious that we will not grasp the subject material, perhaps because this subject seemed difficult in the past. We might already have decided that the subject is dull and, in our view at least, perhaps irrelevant. Rather arrogantly, we might assume that we have already mastered the subject matter and see this as a lecture 'more for those who didn't study this subject previously'. Lectures do not work out exactly as we expect. If we are open to new ideas, we discover something fresh, challenging, interesting and reassuring within most of them. To illustrate this point, imagine the scene where students who hold the assumptions listed in Table 4.1 encounter some rather exciting lectures.

The purpose of Table 4.1 is to highlight how assumptions about a lecture can serve either to enhance or to undermine your learning. If you were the first student, attending a lecture on schizophrenia, you might be delighted to discover that the tutor has adopted such an imaginative approach, introducing you to schizophrenia from the patient's point of view. This is not the usual stance adopted within textbooks. But you will have been jolted from your anticipated line of thought – one that catalogued the signs, symptoms and theories about the condition. Entering this lecture with rigidly set ideas about what will happen next could leave you needing to adjust during the first ten minutes of the presentation.

Lecture subject matter	Student expectation	Lecture format
Understanding mental illness: an introduction to schizophrenia	This lecture will augment what I have read in a textbook (so this is not that valuable)	The lecturer uses a series of audiotapes that first simulate what it is like for patients to 'hear voices' and to suffer delusional thoughts, before discussing a videotape of a patient talking about coping with this.
Risk assessment and management in clinical areas	This is important stuff, but I guess it will list what we have to do, and what we must control or avoid (it will instruct)	The lecturer confronts the audience with a story of a 'near miss' drug error and casts them as fellow investigators in what needs to be done next.
A physiology lesson on endocrine control of the body	I have studied physiology at college before and can list all the important endocrine organs and hormones	The lecturer presents complex information from the start of the lecture. Each student is provided with an electronic device that they can press to indicate when they do not understand something. Lights relating to this show up on the lectern that the lecturer speaks from. The lecturer proceeds apace, provided that lights do not go on in front of him.

Table 4.1: Student expectations and lecture encounters

If you were the second student, you might have been surprised to find that you were cast in the role of fellow incident investigator. The tutor punctuates her lecture with a series of questions to the audience: 'What might we do here?' 'Why do you think this is important?' If you were the third student, your view of your own understanding of endocrinology may have been tested but will you press the button to indicate when you do not understand something that has been said by the tutor? The discomfort of discovering what you really do not know and thought that you did, may mean that you are reluctant to signal to the lecturer that he is covering ground too quickly.

The key point here is that lectures do more than simply convey information (Lancaster et al., 2012). Tutors have become more artful about lecture format, so you need to engage much more carefully with what is shared. Many of the best lecturers collate an eclectic mixture of visual resources, film clips, case studies, debates on the internet and then role model ways in which issues might be considered and problems identified. The virtual and the physical classroom converge.

The best way to prepare mentally for lectures, then, is to acknowledge in advance your misgivings and anxieties, to note perhaps too some prejudices and premises but to approach lectures with a sense of excitement too. Be prepared to applaud innovative teaching, especially that which allows you to better understand how the lecturer interprets and combines information. The lecturer is not only a conveyer of information; he or she is an illustrator of reasoning.

Engaging with the lecture

As we have seen in Table 4.1, lectures may take different forms and they are by no means always dry presentations. Tutors find imaginative ways to interact with students. For example, we have used multi-coloured cubes placed before each student in the lecture theatre, enabling the group as a whole to respond to periodic questions that we pose. We ask students to respond using the different coloured faces of their cubes. Each colour corresponds to an answer from a series of options that appear on the presentation screen. In a lecture on healthcare policy implementation, we might ask the audience which of six options best describes who should be consulted on making the policy work. Perhaps some students show a red face (indicating the healthcare team) and others a yellow face (senior healthcare managers). We hope, though, that most will show the green face of the cube (healthcare teams, managers, patients and lay carers). The tutor is then able both to understand what the students think and to question with them why particular choices have been made.

Engagement, however, is not limited to responding to tutors' questions. It involves attending to the lecture in different ways at different points. Successful students listen with a purpose. De Bono (2009), in a famous account of different ways of thinking, referred to six differently coloured hats that related to the nature of thinking that people might usefully engage in. Each of the metaphorical coloured hats described a different way of attending to what was being said.

- **White hat thinking** focuses upon the data, the facts and the figures. White hat thinking is concerned with evidence and involves the thinker in questions about what we already know. What is already clear in this data and what don't we yet know? White hat thinking is very important, for instance, when we consider statistics. What do experts think the incidence of hospital admissions linked to a pandemic infection might be?

- **Red hat thinking** is concerned with intuition, feelings, emotions and experience. Aspects of nursing care have the potential to evoke strong emotions within us and to reveal, through these, things about our values and beliefs. In a lecture on nursing ethics where case studies are presented, you might need to attend to the feelings evoked.

- **Black hat thinking** describes a more cautious and judgemental form of thinking. It engages the thinker in a debate about whether arguments can be supported. It is not assumed that you will leave every lecture agreeing with the tutor. Indeed, in many instances, the lecture will have served to highlight what your alternative account of matters might be and to prompt reflections on what evidence supports each view.

- **Yellow hat thinking** refers to logical reasoning and especially that which concerns whether something will work. You might use this sort of reasoning in association with theories presented within the lecture. Can these be applied in practice and, if so, to what extent? If a theory–practice gap exists, how big is this and why does it arise?

- **Green hat thinking** is the sort that demonstrates your creativity. It involves you in proposing new ideas and suggestions. In a lecture, it might prove to be important when the tutor invites you to speculate about an ideal form of care delivery or a better way to run a service.

- **Blue hat thinking** refers to what we have previously called metacognition, and engages you in a review of the process of what is going on here. In a lecture, it might be used to sit back and to reflect on the direction in which a debate about vaccination programmes is going. What are we in fact doing here, agreeing there?

Black and yellow hat thinking are especially important with regard to your future written work, where you will be expected to demonstrate your own powers of reasoning. If you sit passively within a lecture and fail to interrogate what the lecturer claims, you are much more likely to adopt a passive approach in your writing too. There is a risk that you will espouse the ideas of your lecturer, rather than your own. Your written work may become descriptive, simply repeating the points that have been lectured to you. While it is unproductive and rude to contest every point with the lecturer on a subject, raising queries in at least some areas both tells him or her that you are being attentive and exercises your own powers of reasoning. Discussion with your lecturer, and possibly with other students, deepens your understanding of key issues. It may certainly help you to remember points that could be raised later in a piece of coursework. It is in teaching sessions such as lectures that you learn to enquire and in some measure, depending on the format of the lecture, to question and debate. Remember, in Table 3.1 (pages 48–9), higher levels of critical thinking are associated with asking how arguments fit with contexts. So asking questions such as whether the espoused ideas work in practice is extremely important. It is necessary to ask yourself, and perhaps the lecturers too, what conditions would have to prevail before an argument made were true? Imagine that your lecturer was sharing with you some of the rights that she believes underpin nursing care. The patient has a right to confidentiality – but you remember that care is often delivered in communal environments where medical rounds are completed. So a question about possible challenges and compromises to the right of confidentiality is entirely reasonable. 'I noted your points about confidentiality, and can see that with regard to patient records. But what about medical rounds and the discussion of problems at the bedside. Is this a problem?'

Raising queries about what a lecturer has said, asking for clarification, is not the mark of an awkward student: instead, queries signal an inquisitive learner. While a lecturer has a number of points that they wish to convey in the time available, they also want the student to learn how to argue. So critical evaluation of points made by lecturers is part of what is required when you attend lectures. Students are not empty receptacles into which lecturers pour information. Lecturers understand and hope that you will process the information too, checking the fit of the new information received with understanding to date.

Blue hat thinking relates closely to reflective practice. We need to ruminate on what has been said by the lecturer. Once again, if you are ready to explore how the claims made by the lecturer affect your current values, beliefs and attitudes, you are beginning to engage with the highest possible level of reflective thinking described in Table 3.2 (pages 50–1). Imagine that the lecturer, in answer to the last student question, contends that nurses of necessity have to compromise sometimes on confidentiality, and that medical rounds on a ward illustrate this. How does that make you feel? Perhaps it seems a 'cop out' and that more medical matters could be covered in a case-notes round away from the bedside. Perhaps you think that significant and intimate information can and should be discussed elsewhere, moving mobile patients to a consultation room.

As you ponder these concerns you deal with your values and the extent to which you think that you can compromise them, the extent to which you might advocate new practice to secure a better standard of practice.

Activity 4.2   *Reflection*

Think back to a lecture that you have attended, one that seemed to challenge you to wear different thinking hats. How much did you learn from that lecture? Did the engagement of your emotions as you reflected during the lecture trigger higher level thinking? If so, how did you follow up afterwards, by visiting the lecturer to discuss points, by enquiring further in the literature?

While the structure and format of a lecture are limited only by the imagination of the tutor and the need to secure particular learning objectives, there are some classic features of most lectures to which we can apply the different thinking hats. In doing this, you are a strategist, switching the way in which you think to suit the different features of the lecture that you come across. The better strategist you become, the more you will be able to integrate learning here to that which you do within other parts of your course; for example, asking questions about how clinical experiences and lecture messages mutually reinforce one another and give you the confidence to practise in a particular way.

Typically a lecture will include:

- **scene-setting and context-relating** – the tutor asks students to focus on a particular subject matter, often linked to lecture goals or objectives;

- **exposition** – where the tutor summarises points discovered through research, presented as theory or indicated by experience; exposition is typically happening when the tutor refers to the literature or states a particular theory;

- **illustration** – tutors sometimes draw on their own personal experience of nursing or that shared by other practitioners;

- **speculation** – where the tutor debates issues or different expositions; for example, two or more theories of counselling may have been shared and the tutor considers the relative merits of each;

- **interrogation and consultation** – where the tutor invites responses from students, either to check their understanding or to engage them further in the subject matter; dependent on the audience size there may be scope for limited group activity;

- **summation** – where the tutor sums up what the lecture has conveyed;

- **next direction** – where the tutor suggests what further work, reading or reflection is now useful.

We can link the different elements of a lecture to the thinking hats that you might need to use, as in Table 4.2.

Features of the lecture	Possible thinking hats
1. Scene-setting and context-relating	a. White hat: focusing on the facts or figures – what do we know and what do we not know?
2. Exposition	b. Red hat: intuition, feelings and emotions
3. Illustration	c. Black hat: caution and judgement
4. Speculation	d. Yellow hat: thinking about the practicalities
5. Interrogation and consultation	e. Green hat: creativity
6. Summation	f. Blue hat: stepping back; what is happening in this lecture, where are we going?
7. Next direction	

Table 4.2: Ways of attending to lecture content

Listening and making notes

To think in the above ways, quizzically and reflectively, testing your own assumptions and those of others, is only possible if you are able to listen attentively. Many students report difficulties with this, as they explain that they are busily writing down information that the tutor has shared. Attending a lecture is seen as an information-gathering expedition and the student then erroneously believes that, because they have amassed a set of notes, they have learnt successfully. It is our experience that, in making extensive notes, there is little scope for the depth or the quality of thinking that helps students to master new subjects or to develop analytical ways of proceeding. A balance needs to be struck between making sufficient notes to aid memory and to prompt activities post-lecture (perhaps writing an assignment), and immersing yourself in the subject of the lecture, thinking carefully about what the tutor says (Berry, 2011). Your understanding may be better facilitated where you have examined the lecturer's points in some depth. So it is often better to make fewer notes and listen more critically to what is said. This is especially true if, as a matter of routine, lecturers make their presentation available within the course intranet.

Activity 4.3   *Critical thinking*

Put your metaphorical black thinking hat on and decide whether you support the above argument about intensive note-taking and the limitations that this sets on thinking in lectures. If you support our argument, consider how you will negotiate handout arrangements with your tutors. If you disagree, what is it about your note-taking that permits you to think deeply as you write?

We do not propose an answer to this activity because it serves simply to help you think about what works for you. We suggest, though, that in more complex and unfamiliar subjects, thinking time within the lecture is vital.

The notes that you do make within a lecture should be sufficient to remind you what was said, in order to trigger later reflections and aid revision. It is unrealistic to write extensive notes at the pace that lectures proceed and to try to do so will leave you frustrated at what you missed. Your notes, then, should be rather like those of a sports journalist who is reporting from a football match – representing events but still allowing you to attend to the new things that you are seeing and hearing. Three of the techniques that you might use include the following.

- Simply list key words or short phrases that capture the essential features of the subject – so much the better if you add exclamation marks or question marks to remind you about what was surprising or seemed questionable. For these to work, you need to commit to 'writing up notes' as soon as possible after the lecture.

- A variant of this is to use a spider diagram, by placing the key concepts centre stage on a piece of paper and then adding branches of related ideas or points, using arrows to show what leads to what and what interacts with other things (see Figure 4.1).

- Summarise only that evidence, or this theory, that the discussion then proceeds from. You will recall the debates afterwards and can add some further points that emerge as you reflect on the lecture afterwards.

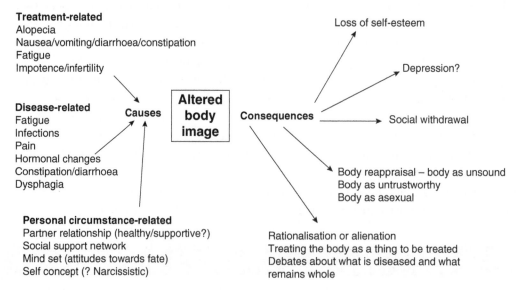

Figure 4.1: Illustration of a spider diagram relating to part of a lecture on altered body image in cancer

The use of questions to facilitate learning

Questions feature regularly within lectures, although many students worry about these. They fear that a question posed by the tutor will seem unanswerable and that, in not venturing an answer or offering the wrong answer, their reputation will be blemished. They are concerned, too, that to ask questions of the tutor may also signal their ignorance, either because the question may seem naive to others or because they fear that the tutor may judge their question as being in some sense inappropriate. You will only develop your critical thinking abilities, however, if you are prepared to engage in questions, asking your own and answering those of your tutor or colleagues. Questions enable you to fill in gaps in your knowledge and to ascertain whether your current grasp of a subject is complete. Tutors know that it feels daunting for a student to engage in questioning, so they use a technique that allows the more confident students to venture answers to questions first. As you attend your next lecture, notice how the tutor poses a question first to the whole group, inviting possible answers from students. The tutor 'poses' the question, then 'pauses', allowing time for everyone to give the question due consideration, and then 'pounces'. If 'pounce' sounds rather intimidating, remember that pose/pause/pounce is simply an aide memoire for teachers learning their craft. The pounce usually involves inviting a student who has signalled interest in answering to proceed with their point. Tutors are taught *not* to embarrass individual students in the class. Where your answer is incomplete, you will usually be congratulated on the successful part of the answer before the tutor invites others to add to it. 'Gina has given us part of the answer here; who can add some more?'

Posing your own questions requires a little thought. It is important to configure a question that is comprehensible to the tutor – one on which others too might perhaps wish to hear an answer – and to ensure that this is a question and not a comment. Students frequently mix up the two, leaving the tutor unsure how best to respond or, at worst, to feel that their teaching has been undermined. In the meantime, you may sound confused to your colleagues, or perhaps opinionated. Here is Stewart, posing a very successful question associated with the lecture on cancer and altered body image:

I was interested in the points that you made about the sort of cancer that patients have and the effect of this on their body image. Some tumours are especially threatening. I've recently nursed a man who had a mouth cancer and he has had to have radical surgery. I wondered whether cancers that affect the face are more distressing?

In this example, Stewart does three things. First, he orientates the tutor to where his question is focused: 'I was interested in the points that you made about …'. Second, he gives the briefest rationale for posing the question: 'I've recently nursed a man …'. Then he poses the question itself: 'I wondered whether …'. Stewart may already have a good idea that patients with head and neck cancers suffer a higher incidence of altered body image. He has witnessed their distress. But he still manages to phrase this as a question that the tutor can answer and others can understand. Had he wished to venture a tentative opinion, and had invited the tutor to either support or disagree with him, the question could have been posed differently:

I have just finished a placement on the head and neck cancer unit and nurses there seem to deal with a lot of psychological distress in patients with facial cancers. This seemed to be because the face is so important for the patient's personal identity and I wondered whether you agree?

As you look at the above offerings from Stewart, you might usefully reflect that the first is the more traditional question. Here, Stewart does not expose so much of his own thinking and it is a good way forward if you feel less sure about the subject of the lecture. If you were feeling more confident and wished to check your understanding, the second approach would be a reasonable and clear way to present the question.

Activity 4.4   *Reflection*

In the next lecture that you attend, pay particular attention to the ways in which questions are posed by students – those who ask for an answer and those who help the individual to check the reasonableness of their ideas. Does the quality of questioning significantly enhance what you take away from a lecture? What do you think that the student who asks questions takes away from the session that other students might not?

After the lecture has finished

Irrespective of whether you made extensive notes within a lecture or whether you answered or ventured questions of your own, we would encourage you not to leave the lecture to one side after it has finished. If it is to make a coherent contribution to the rest of your studies, there are some things that you can do immediately afterwards that will not only reinforce your learning but will also help to motivate your next enquiries as well. Here is our 'to do' list.

- Expand on your notes in order to produce a resource that can assist you with assessments that might lay special emphasis on the command of facts. You may need to consult a textbook to clarify your thinking at this point. Writing points out as paragraphs forces you to express your reasoning in ways that lists cannot. Remember, back in Chapter 3 we highlighted the value of speculation as part of higher level critical thinking, so do not be afraid to include questions and possible ideas about what might be important, what might be happening in your notes. If you prefer, make those points in a different-coloured ink so that you can find them again when further teaching or clinical experience enables you to check your ideas, those embryonic theories, further.

- Identify any things that you do not understand. Where will you find fuller explanations? Perhaps this is something that will be available through a discussion in your personal tutor group. It is unwise to assume that a lecture will have explained everything and that you will be left query free. Recognising what you do not yet know is part of that which drives future learning. You need to understand what knowledge or insight gaps you still have. This is not shameful, it is part of strategic enquiry.

- Make a reflective note concerning your perceptions at this point. If you found some of the arguments made by the tutor unsettling or startling, determine why this is. What within your past experience, attitudes or values led you to alternative perspectives? What, if anything, needs to change now? Now is a good time to commit your reflections to your portfolio and to consider whether you need to discuss any insights that you may have with others.

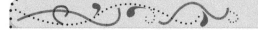

Chapter summary

The lecture is probably the learning opportunity that students think they know the most about and sometimes learn least from. Over-exposure to lectures and making assumptions that one can get by simply by 'listening in' to the key points can undermine what can be

continued ...

achieved by full engagement with a lecture. Lectures are a common feature within nursing courses, so it is foolish not to derive the maximum benefit from them. By engaging with the lecture and its subject matter, you can not only learn a great deal but you can also contribute to the successful learning of others. This chapter has highlighted ways in which different sorts of thinking can relate to different features of the lecture, and how questions that you then pose as well as answer materially enrich everyone's learning. Critically evaluating what the lecturer says exercises you in the sort of higher level thinking that will be valued by assessors in your coursework later.

Preparing carefully for the lecture and following up with reflective notes will significantly enhance what you learn. Materially, though, it is perhaps the quality of thinking within the lecture that determines whether you will develop the inquisitive attitudes that are so important in nursing. In the lecture, you witness the reasoning of another – the tutor. In the years that follow, opportunities to attend lectures, and to witness reasoning writ large, will be few. Learning to use such opportunities now will equip you to go on learning, within your current course and throughout your career.

Further reading

Butterworth, J and Thwaites, G (2013) *Thinking Skills: Critical thinking and problem solving*. Cambridge: Cambridge University Press.

One of the key uses of lectures in senior nurse training is the analysis of problems, the investigation of risk or of management challenges, when no easy solution is available. It seems a good idea to go prepared to such sessions with a good understanding of the nature of problems and their analysis. Unit 3 in this textbook does just that. While the text is not applied to nursing, the evaluative principles remain and you will feel better equipped to engage in debate having read a unit such as this.

Race, P (2014) *Making Learning Happen: A guide to post-compulsory education*. London: Sage.

Professor Phil Race is one of the most enthusiastic, 'can do', 'what about thinking of it this way ...' authors working in education, so we have no reservations recommending this book to nurse teachers who wish to freshen up their teaching approach. It is also worth dipping into for nurse learners, especially when evaluating modules of study and the quality of teaching received.

Walker, A (2015) *Accelerated Learning: Proven accelerated learning techniques to learn more, improve your memory and process information faster*. CreateSpace Independent Publishing Platform.

We have significant reservations about quick fix, trick ways, to learn better. That said, this 36-page booklet is a modest investment to make. It does offer useful material on mind mapping and the use of mnemonic devices that should be of use to you in your studies. Nurses do have to memorise a significant amount of information still, especially in areas such as physiology.

Useful websites

www.humanities.manchester.ac.uk/studyskills/essentials/note-taking/different_models.html

Different models of note-taking

This short summary page is worth visiting if you would like a suggestion on how to set out your note pages in lectures. The Cornell Note Taking System sets out a structure for key words, summaries and issues and questions that occur to you as the lecture progresses. It is a good example of brief note-making procedure.

owll.massey.ac.nz/study-skills/note-taking-methods.php

Note-taking methods

Again, this is a short page summary of note-making options but, if you like the idea of the Cornell Note Taking System referred to above in the Manchester University humanities site, then this site from Massey University offers an example of what that looks like on the page.

http://eprints.lse.ac.uk/50929

Karnad, A (2013) Student use of recorded lectures: a report reviewing recent research into the use of lecture capture technology in higher education, and its impact on teaching methods and attendance. London: London School of Economics and Political Science.

Increasingly lecturers are recording their lectures either as an aid to student revision or so as to increase the number of students who can access their teaching. This short report from LSE Research Online examines what happens when lecturers do this, specifically, whether it changes attendance at live lectures and/or the pattern of student study. We think this a good review for nurse teachers to read, and helpful for learners too.

| Additional Online Material | For examples of analytical essays and other useful material, please visit the companion website at **www.sagepub.co.uk/price_harrington** |

Chapter 5
Making sense of demonstrations, seminars and workshops

....
: ⌇⌇⌇⌇   **NMC Standards for Pre-registration Nursing Education** :
....

This chapter addresses the following competencies.

Domain 1: Professional values

6. All nurses must understand the roles and responsibilities of other health and social care professionals, and seek to work with them collaboratively for the benefit of all who need care.

Domain 2: Communication and interpersonal skills

4. All nurses must use effective communication strategies and negotiation techniques to achieve best outcomes, respecting the dignity and human rights of all concerned. They must know when to consult a third party and how to make referrals for advocacy, mediation or arbitration.

Domain 4: Leadership, management and team working

6. All nurses must work independently as well as in teams. They must be able to take the lead in coordinating, delegating and supervising care safely, managing risk and remaining accountable for the care given.

7. All nurses must work effectively across professional and agency boundaries, actively involving and respecting others' contributions to integrated person-centred care. They must know when and how to communicate with and refer to other professionals and agencies in order to respect the choices of service users and others, promoting shared decision making, to deliver positive outcomes and to coordinate smooth, effective transition within and between services and agencies.

Chapter aims

After reading this chapter, you will be able to:

- describe the key features of a demonstration, a seminar and a workshop;
- indicate how you need to prepare for and attend to the different learning opportunities offered there;
- contrast learning in these settings with that in the lecture.

Introduction

Some of the most influential learning within your course of studies is likely to result from a demonstration, a seminar or one of the several forms of workshop with which you might become involved. The required level of student engagement here (thinking, reflecting, debating, trying out ideas, listening to colleagues) is high, so you will need to be very alert. You will learn within a smaller group, perhaps 10–12 people, and this provides rich opportunities to debate and examine in a way the lecture cannot easily replicate. It is within seminars and workshops in particular that you will learn some of the higher level critical thinking that you first met in Table 3.1 (pages 48–9). Whereas the asking of questions in a lecture might focus on quite general and theoretical points, in seminars and workshops you are dealing with more applied information. You and your colleagues have gathered the information from different places and none of it is necessarily 'tutor sanctioned'. You must judge its merits; your tutor has not interpreted it for you, so you will need to ask questions about its credibility and its fit to the purpose of your seminar or workshop. You will learn to combine a mixture of information, which may be of different types (Pilcher, 2014). There may be information about what is working (perhaps an audit), there may be ethical information (about that which is morally defensible) and research information about cause-and-effect relationships in health care. As part of your group activity, you will need to weigh the merit of these sources of information and to discern what can be concluded from the body of information as a whole. You are much more likely to develop higher level skills in asking questions, discriminating between claims, interpreting and speculating about information, and making arguments where you have to gather and process the information for yourself; all these skills are important to leadership (Buckwell-Nutt et al., 2014). Active engagement in this work is thus critically important.

The often-heard aphorism, 'what I see or hear I forget; what I do, I remember', is true in our experience. Learning in these sessions involves significant student participation and this is usually combined with a less directive, more facilitative role for the tutor (Lucas, 2009). Instead of teaching you the subject, the tutor aids your discovery of it. Learning is likely to be inductive (whereby you create explanations for what is experienced) and deductive (where you then take an emergent explanation and see if that fits with other contexts as well).

Learning from demonstrations

Demonstrations are used to teach you the sort of psychomotor (practical) and interpersonal skills that are so important in nursing (McNett, 2012). While many of these skills are refined within the practice setting, they may be first introduced, on campus, within a skills laboratory or a classroom role play (Hamilton et al., 2014). While learning skills on campus may seem less authentic, it is also less threatening. Your 'patient' may be a manikin designed to provide you with feedback on whether you are proceeding correctly. Manikins do not suffer from less-adept injection techniques, they do not feel pain and they do not become aggressive. There are fewer risks to worry about here. The learning is simulation based and, to facilitate this, your tutor might use a case scenario or might program the manikin to present physical signs or problems in a particular way. Just how sophisticated this becomes depends upon the facilities available within the skills laboratory.

Skill demonstrations often centre on the learning of a particular procedure (e.g., catheterising a patient, giving an injection). But they may also be associated with the interpretation and management of events where there is no set procedure and where the nurse has to respond to a situation moment by moment (e.g., aggressive patients). In the second of these cases, role play may be involved, where you and colleagues are asked to adopt different personae and to act out some possible scenarios (Schlegel et al., 2012). In role play, the tutor's demonstration of what might work best will be offered later on in the session, perhaps improving upon your first efforts. In a demonstration associated with a set procedure, it is likely to be shared first.

Watching a demonstration first provides an excellent opportunity for you to interpret information in a more manageable way. You may, for instance, be able to concentrate on the way in which blood flow either increases or decreases from the manikin's heart, depending on how compressions are managed in a cardiac resuscitation stimulation. The attached monitor enables you to link action (cardiac compressions) to cardiac output in a way that no other teaching method can. A good demonstration helps to de-clutter the information you might otherwise have to process all at once in a clinical situation. You can concentrate on one element of information and, of course, if the demonstration was video recorded, you can run it again and again.

The demonstration of a procedure begins with some briefing about when and why the chosen procedure is used. The tutor then demonstrates the procedure in full, explaining what they are thinking and doing as they go (the overview). Understanding the procedure as a whole is important, as patients experience it this way, as an event. You will usually have to explain the procedure as a whole to the patient before you begin. Procedures are some of the units in which patients evaluate nursing care. A patient might observe, for example, that a particular nurse is very good at 'taking blood'. Afterwards, the overview is broken down into its constituent stages and you are asked to analyse with the tutor what each of those stages involves. Breaking the procedure down into its constituent stages enables you not only to determine what must be done but also to examine why it is done in a particular order or way. You might make use of video footage to examine the procedure in each of its stages. There is an opportunity to ask questions about the procedure and,

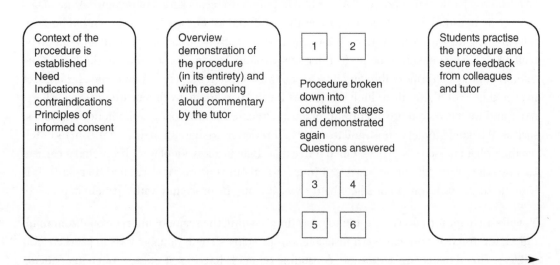

Figure 5.1: Classic procedure demonstration teaching

afterwards, you will be invited to complete the procedure yourself, usually with one or more colleagues acting as reviewers or assistants. The critique of what then proceeded well, and what was less accomplished, is as important as what you learn by watching what the tutor does. Figure 5.1 summarises the steps.

Activity 5.1   *Critical thinking*

Picture a psychomotor procedure of your choice and then decide how the organisation of this procedure in an orderly way might affect whether the nurse then seems compassionate and skilful to the patient. Why is it important to understand the preparation of the patient first? Does the breaking down of a skill help you to understand how physical and psychological care are combined?

Watching an experienced tutor demonstrate a procedure to perfection can seem rather demoralising, but you need to remember just how much practice experience this nurse has. What is at issue here is not whether you can do it as well as them, but whether you understand how the procedure is done, why it is done in a particular way and what issues need to be considered before you can be deemed competent. A procedure that seems both compassionately arranged and skilful is usually one that proceeds in a clearly reasoned sequence. The nurse has a clear strategy and, at best, it is adjusted to suit the patient's circumstances. The skilful nurse uses their knowledge of the patient's anxieties about injections as part of the preparation before the drug is drawn up and administered for instance. Psychological and physical care is combined. So begin by attending critically to what is said and done. Notice the sequence of work undertaken and how the tutor's rationale illuminates what is being done with the hands. It is very unlikely that you will remember everything said and done in the overview demonstration, so try to grasp the essential points there (e.g., what the tutor is trying to achieve, how they show due concern for the patient) and attend to detail in the stage-by-stage demonstration. Do not be afraid to ask questions, especially those involving the word 'why': 'Why did you pause at that point?'; 'Why is it so important to recheck for a pulse now?' At the stage-by-stage demonstration, it is time to consider the detail and to rehearse in your own mind how you will complete the procedure yourself. Once again, do not assume that your performance has to be faultless. It is very unlikely to be perfect first time around. You may proceed more slowly than the tutor, requiring a little more thinking time as you work through the stages. While some procedures may be time critical, if only to limit discomfort for the patient, many others are not. You will get faster and will become more adept with practice. Prepare for now to ask some honest questions, such as 'What did I forget to do?', and to invite your reviewers to share thoughtful criticism too: 'Tell me then what I missed out; what seemed hurried or done in a less adept way.' If you find a particular procedure very difficult to learn, tell your tutor about your worries privately afterwards. It is better to secure some one-to-one help before you attempt the procedure with a patient in practice.

Not all skill demonstrations are quite so procedural. Within the realm of interpersonal communication, for instance, you may learn instead about principles, some valuable ways to proceed. You will learn about managing aggression, consulting others (what do you think?), referring patients to colleagues, identifying and resolving problems. Demonstration is used here to help you manage some of the uncertainty associated with practice, which can seem 'messy' in nursing. In these demonstrations, work typically begins with a scenario, a clinical problem or need, where different parties might adopt different stances on how best to proceed (e.g., the patient, a relative, the nurse and a doctor). Participants in the role play are given cards describing their roles and some of the things that might reasonably concern them. The cards might suggest what you should hope to achieve. You then begin a period of improvised acting, during which you play your role and respond to others talking or acting towards you. A skilful tutor will allow the role play to develop for several minutes and will then intervene to help you pick out some observations about what was happening, to help you to explore how that felt. Key points might attend to:

- whether the activity was proceeding as you hoped (why or, conversely, why not?);
- whether you felt comfortable with what you were doing or saying;
- whether you felt you understood what another person did or said;
- whether there are other ways in which you could have handled a particular passage of interaction.

When you deliberate on these matters it is worth considering the different levels of critical reflection detailed in Table 3.2 (pages 50–1). Role play sometimes exposes us to some of our own values and beliefs – those that have operated subliminally in our day-to-day lives. Higher level reflection not only attends to possible alternative perspectives on what is happening in the role play, it also attends to what we believe and why those beliefs are valuable or problematic in some way. Imagine, for example, that you see people as rational, health-seeking individuals who do their best to live as sensibly as possible. Now, in the role play, your colleague acting as the patient says to you, 'I won't give up cigarettes, because they help keep me calm. I feel better because of my fags. Besides, if I do, I'll eat too much and die of excess cholesterol!' While the relative risks of cigarettes and cholesterol might be compared statistically, deeper debate centres on whether your working model of how patients should behave is adequate. How will you respond to patients who do not see sensible behaviour in the way that you do?

At intervals in the role play, the tutor may invite some of you to take 'time out' from acting and to watch them manage the interaction for a few minutes. The tutor shows you a different way to converse or different things that could be suggested in the case scenario at this point. Skilful tutors will help you to compare your performance with theirs and, within the supportive setting of your study group, they will encourage you to recount your assumptions about what is right, what seems obvious or logical. If this seems at first uncomfortable, it remains a vital rehearsal for care situations that you might face; for example, in the care of dying patients, decision making in casualty or when dealing with patients who have quite different cultural expectations of good care. Equally importantly, the facilitated discussion confirms to you that you do sometimes need to discuss attitudes and values. These will be important if you are to enter placements and demonstrate practice that seems professional, measured and considerate.

Successful role play can:

- 'inoculate' you against some surprises or discomforts associated with learning in practice. It can help you to deal with the views, reactions and perspectives of others in a more confident way. The investment made here is then a very valuable one. This is your safe place to try out ideas.

- help you to appreciate the artistry and the skill of nursing. Seize the opportunity to ask the tutor about their reasoning. You might not have so much time to discuss reasoning when you are engaged in clinical work yourself.

- help you to appreciate that there is sometimes no perfect way to proceed, only better ways. You learn to respect your own efforts and the value of thinking aloud with others about what you have experienced. You will encounter doubt during your course, so appreciating that more experienced nurses confront this too can be reassuring.

We discussed role play with our four consultant students. Fatima observed that she found it helpful because it assisted her to think through interprofessional relationships. Nurses and other professionals did not necessarily train together and may start with different assumptions that need to be understood. She was relieved we had rehearsed such possibilities before clinical placements. Gina said she saw this learning as vital, because it was what helped her to think about how best to demonstrate compassion. Communication was everything if the patient and relatives were to feel confident regarding what she did. Raymet did not like this form of learning but conceded that some insights gained could not be secured any other way. Stewart enjoyed the learning and wished that similar opportunities had been possible in his previous career. Each of these students has a different learning style and preference, and this might influence how they reacted to role play and demonstrations embedded within that. Some learning sessions would necessarily then seem easier than others.

Activity 5.2   *Reflection*

Look back to Tables 3.1 and 3.2 (pages 48–9 and 50–1) to review which levels of critical thinking and of reflection role play might help you with. Your needs are likely to be individual and dependent, for example, on the stage of your training and your field of practice. Nonetheless, did you find yourself in role play exercising arguments, presenting some of your own and examining those of others? Did you pause to consider whether role play exercises your imagination about how others feel and think, so that you could speculate more about what might happen if you acted in a particular way?

Learning within seminars

Interaction is also equally important in seminars, another form of group learning. In a seminar, individual students are briefed to fulfil different information-gathering tasks within the literature or on the internet and to bring back their discoveries to the group, sharing what they have found and discussing what this might mean with their colleagues (Lorette, 2012). In some instances, the discussion of findings is handled electronically, using a wiki (Morley, 2012). Seminars are typically arranged within a tutorial group, where no more than 10–12 students make a contribution.

Seminars are designed to teach you study skills (especially those relating to search and find), project management skills (you need to work to a common project end) and critical thinking skills – a weighing up of evidence and options available. You will need to be disciplined in your work and brave enough to report your discoveries. Because everyone is asked to contribute in this way, seminars also teach you that you can learn from colleagues as well as a tutor. They help you to develop more collaborative ideas about learning.

Activity 5.3 — *Group work*

As it takes a little while to build confidence as a seminar learner, you might find it useful to practise this work informally with some colleagues before you tackle a bigger exercise within a class. Choose a news story reported in the press, one where a problem seems to exist. If that relates to healthcare, great. Another sort of story, perhaps one about crime, or economic issues, is equally useful. Next, each take a different newspaper that reports the story and summarise what is focused upon, how the problem is perceived. Examine how the newspaper report accounts for the problem, why it happened or what seems likely to be at fault. Then report your findings back to an informal student group to gain an understanding of how stories may vary. Did all newspapers identify the same problem? Did some seem to suggest that there was no problem at all, or else that the origin of the problem came from somewhere quite different? This is what a seminar involves, the gathering and critical comparison of information. You will share speculative discussions about the subject matter chosen, but also about how this was interpreted by others. The narration as well as the subject matter is important when we apply this work to health care.

During the search stage of any seminar work, you will need to find the best possible paper, website or clinical insight to share. If you bring back something that is not so well thought through, which is not quite clear, more discussion work will be needed at the end. There is a gentle element of competition here, as each group member should try to secure the best possible, most informative material. During the report and discussion stage of the seminar, it is important to present a clear summary of your discovery and what you make of it. Afterwards you will need to stand ready with constructive questions for those who present their work, for example, 'So how confident do you feel about the author's claims?'; 'Are there situations where these arguments don't hold good?'

Seminar work focuses you, then, firmly on discrimination critical thinking (what material to use, what seems best), on interpretation critical thinking (what the authors are really arguing), on speculative critical thinking (as your group discusses what the significance of this information might be) and on the making of arguments (as you report back to your tutor what you think should now follow). Your tutor is likely to work within the seminar group to help you do a number of things: first, to periodically determine what you seem to be concluding or what you agree for the time being remains uncertain or problematic (summarising); second, they may suggest other questions, alternative perspectives for you all to consider (acting as an agent provocateur); third, the tutor may gently warn you when your discussions are going 'off track', perhaps getting stuck within a blind alley (acting as a guide). The contributions that they make, though, will often remain speculative in nature. The tutor will be at pains not to instruct you. Were they to do so, the seminar would quickly change into a teaching session and you would be tempted to make your presentation not to the group but to the tutor. Anticipate that, during seminar sessions, tutor input will often be less directive in nature. Your tutor is not simply playing games with you but is facilitating different forms of learning that foster self and collective group reliance.

Learning within workshops

Among the workshops that you might be invited to take part in are the following.

- **Masterclasses** – an expert practitioner helps you to rehearse your practice skills. Masterclasses combine demonstration with guidance and feedback as you attempt to emulate practice. Supportive feedback on your performance is encouraged from the rest of the study group. Example: listening techniques to assist anxious patients.

- **Problem-based learning sessions** (Spiers et al., 2014) – these are typically based on patient-care scenarios. You and your colleagues are invited to use available evidence to work out what the important issues are, what is problematic and how you will then proceed. Example: managing a patient's chronic pain.

- **Journal clubs** – you agree a collective reading strategy that acquaints you with the facilities of the library and prepares you for the day, post-registration, when you will make continuing use of journals to update your practice (Dovi, 2015). You review a sequence of found articles, everyone reading the same work to concentrate the analysis shared. Example: critical review of different research designs.

This is a just a selection. Your teachers may suggest others.

Workshops are important in nursing curricula because, as a healthcare professional, you will later be charged with collaborating with colleagues to achieve goals. If your studies solely consisted of lectures and clinical practice, it would be much more difficult for you to develop a more independent and collegiate form of learning.

Workshops, then, are not as one student once suggested: a means for the tutor to gain some respite from teaching. They are carefully structured activities that require the tutor to help you to develop more independent enquiry. Some of the things that facilitate learning here are under the tutor's control, while others are under your control. Good workshop design is the work of the tutor.

Working with others to manage uncertainty within the workshop group is your responsibility. You will need to set aside the notion that colleagues cannot teach you as well as the tutor and examine what collective experience offers. We suggest that working towards a discernible product at the end of your workshop helps bring purpose to your work.

Where students typically report problems with workshop learning, it is usually because of one or more of three things. First, the learning seemed more arduous and less time-efficient than if a conventional lecture had been used. Students wondered what had been achieved there that could not have been done so using another learning method. A lack of insight into the purpose of workshops thwarted progress. Second, one or more people within the learning group undermined the project work being completed. Colleagues may have baulked at the work required and not contributed a fair share of effort. Third, the project seemed poorly structured and managed. Colleagues felt that they were left for too long to wonder and debate about an issue, when the group suspected that the tutor knew the answers anyway and could have been rather more supportive.

Activity 5.4 — *Reflection*

Take a moment to reflect on any workshops that you have been involved in, and to determine whether they seemed successful.

- What did it feel like to learn together as a group?
- If the workshops were successful, what made them so?
- If they seemed wanting in some regard, what seemed to undermine them?

In our experience, where students report successful workshop learning, this is also typically associated with three things. First, there was a sense of achievement linked to the discoveries made, both those that were personal and those that the group managed between them. Second, there was surprise at what was discovered through group work, not merely about the subject of investigation, but about the process of working as a team. Colleagues in these groups noted that the learning was about processes as well as knowledge bases. Third, there was pleasure in working with others, within a group that seemed to 'gel'. Students reported that the purposeful association with others was stimulating and often reassuring in a field of practice that so often seemed to test the individual rather than recognise the work of the group.

In part, then, the success of a workshop is determined by your expectations of learning and their fit (or otherwise) with the requirements of the course. If your learning style is more private, perhaps more passive, and you are receptive and contemplative, rather than strategic and collaborative, workshop learning will seem more difficult. If you are inquisitive and explorative by nature, and enjoy working with others to achieve goals, workshop learning will seem attractive. However, nursing does emphasise team work and collaboration, and learning from experience, so workshops are an important way of learning (see, for example, Zehler (2015), who explains how team support can support casualty nurses through the stresses that they encounter). The ability to develop and then to demonstrate independent thought, right at the top of the critical thinking and reflective reasoning hierarchy, is closely associated with a willingness to learn from colleagues and to collaborate towards shared discoveries.

Managing uncertainty

At the heart of all workshop learning is the need to manage uncertainty. What is required of us, of me, and what shall we do to manage the project set before us? What might be achieved, missed or perhaps misunderstood? What mistakes might happen to confuse our understanding of a subject or perhaps risk a loss of personal reputation, as a student and as a nurse? What might excite and motivate me for the future? If we can manage uncertainty, learning becomes more purposeful and pleasurable.

If, however, the workshop was designed to leave no questions remaining, no enquiries to conduct and no issues to debate, there would be no scope for learning through experience. We would not understand what effort it takes to reach decisions or to make policies or protocols, and we would not understand how groups can operate together to develop strategies of their own. Raymet felt the uncertainty of her group learning activities acutely. She recorded in her portfolio:

> *What alarmed me about the exercises was not only just how much we didn't know. No, what alarmed me was how little there was in this area that offered a right answer, the correct way to act. I craved assurance and only gradually learned to trust my team mates and myself to make good decisions.*

Activity 5.5 — *Critical thinking*

Look at the following list of possible ways of resolving group learning uncertainty and decide which of these could have helped you with past problems encountered while working with others. That experience may come from a past course or outside nursing – the principles still hold good. As you examine these options, reflect on the extent to which each adds clarity of purpose to group working.

- Ask the tutor to clarify the project brief before you set off.
- Check what arrangements are in place for ensuring that work proceeds in the right direction.
- Set out a schedule of work, agreeing what sorts of activity are needed and deciding in what order these will be tackled.
- Agree a means of recording your progress, the decisions that you have made and the discoveries made.
- Determine group etiquette; that is, an agreed way of talking about each other's and colleagues' contributions.

To complete your group activities, it is necessary to start with the clearest possible brief. If yours seems unclear, you should ask the tutor to clarify points for you. In most instances, group activities are supported by a written brief and starter materials. Within a problem-based learning exercise, for example, there is likely to be one or more patient case studies and associated tasks to complete. Typically, too, the project will set out the aims and objectives of the exercise, so that you can sense what work is necessary.

While tutors do not direct the work of the group, they are required to monitor your work. To leave less-experienced nurses without a source of guidance would be both unproductive and demotivating. It is a good idea, then, to check with the tutor when they will intervene to ensure that enquiries continue in an appropriate way. Consulting with the tutor on a regular basis in projects that span several weeks is important. Such 'check points' allow you to ascertain whether work is proceeding towards the required objectives, although your tutor is unlikely to give you a whole 'teaching staff solution'.

Here is a typical response that Raymet received on a problem-based learning exercise:

I think that you're making good progress. The things that you are debating about epilepsy and social stereotypes are exactly what I would think about. But you need to think too about what propels the care plan forward. If worries paralyse you as well as the parents of this child, you won't be serving them very well. Have a think this week about what is known about managing epilepsy.

Project groups are usually composed of students with a mix of aptitudes, and it is certainly not expected that all group members will be good at everything. Indeed, sometimes the tutor devises project groups to help students to explore and share their aptitudes. To gain the benefit of individual aptitudes, however, you will need to be prepared to volunteer what you feel comfortable doing, even if you believe your work might not be perfect. You will also need to acknowledge the work done by others who have other talents. Setting aside personal insecurities is part of the learning process. Start with the assumption that we all have insecurities, many of which are unspoken. What is more important now is that what you share works to achieve project ends. Here is Raymet again:

I'm not imaginative or creative. I could see that Annette and Sean were the creative ones and that was so good. I thought to myself, you must work at this, you cannot rely on just these two. That was why I volunteered to make the notes and to sum up our decisions at different points. I was the scribe of our group and later on that was valuable, as we found so much information it would have been easy to have lost our way.

Wasted time increases the pressures on a group, especially as they near the point where they must present their findings. For that reason, agreeing a schedule of work and how much time is allocated to each part of the project helps to discipline the enquiry.

Instead of a project that finishes with a lot of information about just one thing, you will have a project that seems balanced and measured, professional and insightful. As we have seen above, it is then necessary to keep a brief record of the lines of enquiry and the decisions made. Such an 'audit trail' enables the group to tell the story of their enquiry, as well as to present the end product of what they have learned. What did we consider, what did we conclude, what was left to one side for now, and how did we arrive at our decisions?

Simple group etiquette rules ensure that colleagues are treated with respect and that each contributes in an adequate measure to the work in hand. For example, rules might set out expectations regarding attending meetings, supplying copies of interesting evidence found, and listening attentively until a colleague has presented the whole of their findings. Most project briefs will refer to such group etiquette and either set some parameters for you to follow or suggest which ones need to be agreed.

Creating an end product

Workshop activity prompts you to combine the skills of critical thinking and reflection that have been presented in Part 1 of this book. Because projects change over time, there is a need for reflection. Because projects demand of you decisions and selective use of resources, you have to think critically, discriminating what is worthy of your attention.

Workshop context	Typical end products
Masterclass	A revised demonstration of a skill (e.g., using a manikin simulator, two video records are made of wound-dressing techniques, one before and one after the masterclass; you then invite the audience to make notes comparing the two performances)
Problem-based learning session	An illustrated verbal presentation to the wider group (in some instances more than one group explore the same problem, the better afterwards for everyone to discuss aspects of problem analysis) (e.g., working with families to manage childhood epilepsy)
Journal club	A collaborative, written critique of the chosen papers; the journal papers and their relevant critiques might then be made available through the library for wider consultation and discussion (e.g., a critique of papers that illustrate phenomenological research in nursing; comparisons and conclusions)

Table 5.1: Workshop contexts and typical 'end products'

Project work is not open-ended, and there is a need to reach closure, sharing what you have discovered with others and evaluating what the activity has taught you. It is to this end, to reach a closure that is satisfying and helpful, that nursing courses usually require some sort of 'end product' at the conclusion of the project.

Working towards the workshop end product contributes to your reflective abilities. While workshop activity linked to a long-term project has the greatest potential in this regard, all workshops have the potential to support some reflection. Figure 2.2 (page 32) detailed several benefits of reflection and we see a number of the above end products making a contribution here. These are summarised in Table 5.1.

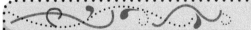 Chapter summary

Demonstrations, seminars and different forms of workshop represent some of the most active learning that you are likely to engage in on your nursing course. The learning is proactive; it requires you to engage carefully with what is required and to contribute questions, ideas and experiences that can mutually advance the learning in hand. While demonstrations might allow a more passive approach, you are most likely to master the skill if you have asked questions during the session. Nursing skills require due consideration of how, why, when and where something is done and you are only likely to understand that if you have discussed the procedure with the nurse who demonstrates it.

continued ...

Seminars and workshops emphasise learning within the group. You will learn as much about the process and enquiry as about the subject matter of the project work shared. You will need to be well organised here, diligent and consultative. Reasoning in these contexts requires more collaboration and effort. It is an investment well made, however. Much of the nursing you will practise later relies upon just such shared learning.

Further reading

Ballett, J and Campling, P (2011) *Intelligent Kindness: Reforming the culture of healthcare.* London: Royal College of Psychiatrists.

Much of what is learned within role play and other forms of workshop learning is designed to improve the emotional intelligence of healthcare staff, to make students more aware of the experiences and needs of others. This book provides a welcome review of why that is important, not just for patients but for more satisfying professional work in the healthcare setting.

Barrett, T and Moore, S (2011) *New Approaches to Problem-Based Learning: Revitalising our practice in higher education.* Abingdon: Routledge.

Although most of the papers within this volume are addressed to academic staff, the first chapter's explanations of problem-based learning and how it operates is good for all. The later sections on expectations of students as learning partners will help you understand what tutors are trying to do when they set up problem-based learning projects.

Cole-King, A and Gilbert, P (2011) Compassionate care: the theory and the reality. *Journal of Holistic Healthcare,* 8(3): 29–37. Available at: www.connectingwithpeople.org/sites/default/files/Compassionate%20 care%20ACK%20and%20PG.pdf

Although this article is a few years old, it is particularly good at exploring what a concept means theoretically and in application. Much of what is harvested for a seminar on nursing care comes from a theoretical stance and the need to demonstrate more compassion in care today prompts us to ask the question, 'How does this translate into something that we must be or show to patients?'

Health and Care Professions Council (2014) *Professionalism in Healthcare Professionals: Research report.* London: HCPC. Available at: www.hpc-uk.org/assets/documents/10003771Professionalisminhealthcare-professionals.pdf

One of the best ways of conducting a seminar is to base it on a new piece of research or a report from a professional body. This one is a very good source example. It explores the way in which professionalism (and its limits) are understood by a range of healthcare professionals regulated by the Council. Nurses have their own code of conduct but it is instructive to see professionalism as it is understood by others.

Skelton, J (2008) *Role Play and Clinical Communication: Learning the game.* Oxford: Radcliffe.

All healthcare students need to hone their communication skills at the bedside and this book offers a critical review of how doctors and their teachers are trying to do that. It is a useful read for nurses, too, as much to help them understand what medical colleagues also wrestle with as to understand the role play approach itself.

Zahavi, D (2014) *Self and Others: Exploring subjectivity, empathy and shame.* Oxford: Oxford University Press.

This textbook will prove a challenging but worthwhile read. At issue first is how well do we know our selves and, if we do not, what capacity can we have to demonstrate empathy? Attention shifts to empathetic relationships, the way expressed empathy might be rewarded within a relationship. While the author does not centre his work on health care as such, it constantly prompts thoughts about care situations, difficult patients and problematic relationships.

Useful website

www.cqc.org.uk/content/compassionate-care

Care Quality Commission

What is quality care and how do patients and relatives see this? How do health and social care professionals understand this concept? This website not only provides you with a link to the UK Chief Nursing Officer's document *Compassion in Practice*, it also affords you the opportunity to join forums on the quality of care. This gives you a chance to see how forums further facilitate critical thinking through review of others' experiences.

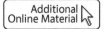

Additional Online Material

For examples of analytical essays and other useful material, please visit the companion website at **www.sagepub.co.uk/price_harrington**

Chapter 6
Making sense of clinical placements

NMC Standards for Pre-registration Nursing Education

This chapter addresses the following competencies.

Domain 1: Professional values

1. All nurses must practise confidently according to *The Code: Professional standards of practice and behaviour for nurses and midwives* (Nursing and Midwifery Council, 2015) and within other recognised ethical and legal frameworks. They must be able to recognise and address ethical challenges relating to people's choices and decision-making about their care, and act within the law to help them and their families and carers find acceptable solutions.

8. All nurses must practise independently, recognising the limits of their competence and knowledge. They must reflect on these limits and seek advice from, or refer to, other professionals where necessary.

Domain 2: Communication and interpersonal skills

1. All nurses must build partnerships and therapeutic relationships through safe, effective and non-discriminatory communication. They must take account of individual differences, capabilities and needs.

2. All nurses must use a range of communication skills and technologies to support person centred care and enhance quality and safety. They must ensure people receive all the information they need in a language and manner that allows them to make informed choices and share decision making.

Chapter aims

After reading this chapter, you will be able to:

- summarise the nature of critical enquiry you need to engage in within clinical placements;
- detail what preparations will enable you to complete a successful clinical placement;
- discuss the part played by the student–mentor relationship in a satisfying and effective learning placement;

(Continued)

(Continued)

- explore the part placement learning plays in the service of more patient-centred care, that which respects the dignity and integrity of others;
- understand the reflective and open approach you must use if feedback is to aid your studies.

Introduction

You are about to venture forth on your first clinical placement. What will it be like? What are the expectations associated with the placement? Will you make mistakes and can the staff tolerate that? Will there be someone there to support you? Irrespective of whether you are now a veteran of many such clinical placements or approaching your first one, the above questions and ones like them are likely to sound familiar. Learning within the clinical setting is exciting but potentially stressful, and it is helpful to understand why that is, and what you can do to counter the anxieties. Clinical placements are where you will have to develop your reflective reasoning abilities. There is little room for absolutist thinking here. The best care is usually nuanced and it is mediated by patient needs and circumstances prevailing. But you will need to think on your feet as you act and then protect some time too to look back and muse on what episodes of care teach you.

In this chapter, we explain what is different about learning in the clinical setting; what you should do when preparing to join a clinical placement; how you might work better with your mentor there; and what might be done to ensure that you do well in clinically based assessments. We pay particular attention to the skills of observation, questioning, interpreting and speculating as they apply here. Critical thinking and reflection have a particular resonance, because of the wealth and diversity of information you will encounter. These skills will play a central role in helping you to both enjoy and learn from the time you spend in the clinical area. We examine how an understanding of narratives and discourses here can help you to develop the sort of empathetic skills that are central to the work of nurses and our reputation with the public at large.

Why clinical learning is different

We asked Gina to make her key points about why clinical learning was different. Here are her observations:

What immediately impressed me was that this was a workplace and that learning had to be much more 'on the hoof'. That shouldn't have surprised me, but honestly, the impact of this change is bigger than you imagine. You forget how centre stage you are in the classroom, how much your learning means to the teaching staff. The clinical staff care, but learning has to fit in with the delivery of services. It's right and proper that the first concern of staff is the patients and the ways in which they experience care.

The second thing I noted was that some of their teaching wasn't about the skill of nursing, it was about the etiquette of practice. I was being socialised into the team and being taught about where, how and when to ask questions. On reflection, that wasn't surprising, as clinical practice is a theatre, it's where the public witness what we do. The staff were anxious about whether I might damage their reputation.

The third thing I noticed was how difficult it was to obtain a rationale for what was being done. You suddenly realise how much trained staff carry in their heads. I felt like a child, always wanting some-one to answer the question 'why?'! Clearly, the nurses couldn't always answer those questions, and especially in front of anxious patients. You had to wait for explanations.

The fourth thing I would say is that you face an information deluge. By that I mean you cannot stop to consider all the options, not as you might wish to anyway. It was the speed of thinking that blew me away and made me wonder whether I would ever learn here.

Gina offers an excellent summary of what makes learning in the clinical environment differ-ent. There is far less structure to the learning experience when compared to a well-run lecture. Students are required to seize the initiative and ask pertinent questions about what is happening. Clinical mentors are mindful not to overestimate students' confidence or ability, but they do not automatically remember to explain points that to them are second nature. Students might be supervised by a range of different people, each with their own way of supporting students (Hasson et al., 2013). There is, then, a need to choose when to ask the right questions, and Gina is right to infer that questions can seem impertinent if asked at the wrong moment. Learning the etiquette of enquiry is important, not only because it helps you to become part of the clinical team, but also because it enables the practitioners to carry on their work.

What Gina's account emphasises is the need to think in an inductive way: 'What is happening here?' Such inductive questions help you make sense of experiences, which is highlighted by Gina as she talks about the speed at which colleagues think. Clinical placements can overload you with informa-tion, and it is not necessarily presented in a coherent form (Cohen, 2013). You are confronted with a series of jigsaw pieces that you will need to fit together to create a picture. Some of those pieces you already have: they come from your past lectures, the theory of nursing and lessons on physiol-ogy, pharmacology and practical skills. Others will become available in placement – those connected with the patients, their diagnoses, their experiences (expressed as stories or narratives) and current treatments. This situation reflects the reality of practice for qualified staff as well. All must continue to make sense of events, and the challenges and needs that arise wherever patients are cared for.

Much of the higher-order reflective reasoning that you read about in Chapter 3 is associated with this sense-making ability. You have to reason contextually. That is, that you have to imagine and speculate about how patients feel, what they know or do not know and what they might most likely want from any care episode that you share. Some of this you learn from accumulating personal experience, what would assure or support you, but much more is learned from listening to what patients hope for. Notice what they say, how they say it and what they chose to focus upon. When they return again and again to the same topics, there are often unresolved concerns worrying them. As you work with patients, you will need to confront that patient's preferences, attitudes, beliefs and values may on occasion be different to yours. So you need to explore their preferences and hold in abeyance sometimes that which you believe to be best, what you would wish to happen to you. The highest level of reflective reasoning operates within the realms of beliefs and values, as well as dealing with the pragmatic circumstances of care delivery (see Table 3.2, pages 50–1).

Thus, to learn effectively in clinical placements you will need to be inquisitive, sensitive to others around you, analytical as you piece together disparate pieces of information, and diligent (Ailey et al., 2015). You will need to deal with a greater level of uncertainty than you may have been accustomed to previously, but you are also likely to be reassured as more experienced nurses describe their own learning curve. One nurse advised Gina:

> *One of the things you learn here is how to build up a picture of what is required by a patient. You learn to accept that you are always learning, always questioning your last ideas. You don't do that on your own; the team help you and expect you to share what you think as the process continues.*

To Gina's list of characteristics of clinical learning, we would add a fifth important point, that learning here is communal. Elsewhere, you may have learned in a more private and personal way. In the clinical arena, there is less scope for private deliberation. The team only learns how best to care for patients if its members share their incremental insights. This is ably illustrated in a number of processes that you will witness, including:

- 'teaching' rounds, where clinicians deliberate on care strategies;

- report handovers, where the team deliberate on the care delivered so far and where new priorities are identified, and on what the patient or relative is saying, which helps explain how they see the situation today and challenges head;

- case conferences, where individual patient care is discussed in some depth and next steps are contemplated.

Practice narratives and discourses

In Chapter 2, we introduced practice narratives – the accounts and discourses that are the focus for a great deal of placement-based learning. We now look at how these are connected to the development of empathy, which is vital in nursing (Atherton and Kyle, 2015). Look back to Table 3.2 (pages 50–1) and note just how much the development of empathy is high-order reflective thinking. To practise empathetically is to demonstrate, at a minimum, contextual level reflection and, at best, independent thinking. Empathetic thinking, understanding and respecting the concerns of others, in the face of your own personal values, demonstrates an extremely high level of professionalism. You will need to be supportive not only of patients and their relatives but also of professional colleagues. Because the clinical environment includes a great deal of uncertainty (what is wrong, what is happening, what might work best, what is safe?), it is especially important to listen hard to what is said and to try to ascertain what is meant. We can illustrate the importance of this by sharing a scenario with you. Imagine a situation where a patient (Mr Jones) has for some weeks suffered from a productive cough. The sputum produced now is bloodstained. The patient, a cigarette smoker in his mid-60s, has recently lost weight. His wife fusses around him while he waits for some tests to confirm the diagnosis.

Mr Jones remarks that the cough is a nuisance and he has lost sleep over it. His back aches and he struggles to inhale deeply. He admits that the cigarettes 'haven't helped'. Of course, the difficulty sleeping might simply be about waking as a result of the cough. But it could also be about anxiety and his fear of what the bloodstained sputum signifies. You will only understand the underlying narrative (his real concerns) if you piece together a collection of things that he has said. You will only learn about this patient's needs and worries if you enquire a little further: 'So how have you been feeling about this?'; 'We must wait for the tests, but I wondered how you prefer to deal with uncertainty?' Here and now, the questions have a particular function, to establish what worries the patient and demonstrate a proper concern for him as a person. You are unable to confirm what is wrong, nor can you pre-empt what senior colleagues will deduce or recommend. It must be enough to understand and, where appropriate, to report on the patient's concerns to others.

Mr Jones, though, is not the only person who is developing a narrative here – an explanatory story of what they think is happening. Mrs Jones and the doctor investigating his problem are also building narratives. Mrs Jones's fussing might simply express love and concern, but it could also relate to past knowledge of what bloodstained sputum could mean. Her father died of tuberculosis and he showed similar signs. You will only understand and support Mrs Jones if you are able to learn a little more about this narrative from what she hints at, and what she begins to signal through her care activities. 'My husband always tries to see the positive in everything, but I know that things don't always turn out so well,' she said, and this is an opportunity to gently enquire further.

The doctor's account of events can be described as scientific and investigative. He has begun a methodical series of investigations to help confirm one diagnosis and to exclude others. His accounts, especially before the patient, are measured and cautious; he does not wish to reach any premature conclusions. But if you have the opportunity to ask him, and talk about what he sees and hears, you might learn that his narrative is about the possibility of lung cancer. He may express all the same concerns that you feel. But you can only help manage communication and patient support before diagnosis (the discourse under way) if you hear what he says.

What is important, then, is that you listen with purpose and attend carefully. An understanding of the narratives will help you to ask appropriate questions at the appropriate times. You realise it is necessary to understand the doctor's deliberations before you venture into more extensive discussions with the patient. If you inadvertently lead the patient to premature conclusions, possibly the wrong ones, the work of the healthcare team may be more difficult. So you search for patterns of information. These tests (for cells within the sputum, a bronchoscopy and the detailed notes within the patient history taken) suggest the possibility of lung cancer. They alert you to the importance of understanding the patient's worries, without, at this stage, alarming him. The balance of listening and explaining is determined by your reading of the situation. Remember, just because your coping style is to have all the possible diagnoses spelled out from the outset, the patient's coping style might not be. Rational insight guides your thinking, how you see yourself as a person, but it might be very different for Mr Jones. Before a diagnosis is confirmed, listening and understanding are key. After a diagnosis, the emphasis may shift to explaining and reassuring. Where you clearly attend to the concerns of the patient or relative, listening hard and clarifying what worries them, you demonstrate compassion. It is not assumed that you will automatically and instantly resolve patients' difficulties, but you will establish a reputation for treating them as individuals.

Activity 6.1   *Reflection*

Look back to Gina's four points regarding what makes clinical learning different and draw upon any personal experience gained so far to illustrate these in action. For example, can you cite examples of where you think you were being socialised into the clinical team? Next, study the points above regarding accounts, narratives and discourses. Can you recall any clinical placement incidents that confirm the importance of attentive listening, identifying the narratives and the discourses that underpin what is said or done there?

Preparing for the placement

Preparation for your placement can significantly reduce the anxiety that you feel on your first days there. The more you can bring structure and order to the learning experience, working with your mentor, the more constructive the learning will seem. Table 6.1 suggests what might be done in advance of your placement.

Strategy	Benefit
Review the learning outcomes that have to be achieved during this placement and any assessment arrangements that apply.	You focus on what has to be achieved.
Research the work of the department, ward or practice by looking at any details on healthcare agency websites and by asking students who have had placements there before.	By asking some preliminary questions you won't have to ask quite so many on your placement. Interpreting what is going on will seem easier.
Revisit your portfolio to identify particular practice skills that you like wish to improve on, for example patient history taking.	You calmly discriminate what needs your attention. Explaining where you would particular guidance helps the mentor to plan their support.
Make personal contact with the clinical team, writing or emailing the nurse in charge.	You establish an immediate rapport if you show such personal organisation. You make your first argument: I am diligent and well prepared and I value this placement.
Try to establish in advance who your mentor will be.	Knowing this, and whether you might share the same shift, will increase your confidence and is one less thing to think about later. Successful mentors' reputations sometimes go before them.

Strategy	Benefit
Ascertain what sorts of illness, injury or other health challenge are confronted by patients in this clinical area. Make a note of what might worry them most and what might seem most sensitive as regards communication there. For example, if patients are suffering from cancer, the management of information pre-diagnosis is of great concern. Patients may be especially concerned about prognosis or the effects of treatment. Jot them down. Check when your first shift is and arrive in good time, correctly attired.	By anticipating what may be of greatest concern and require the most careful enquiry, you can demonstrate to your mentor at first interview that you have a due concern for both patients and colleagues. You start well.

Table 6.1: Getting ready for clinical placement study

Activity 6.2   *Reflection*

Refer to your portfolio and check whether there are practice skills that you promised to focus on in your next clinical placement. If not, write in your portfolio three skills that you wish to develop further, adding a short rationale to each. Referring to these skills in your first conversation with your mentor will demonstrate your commitment and personal organisation. You are likely to get more from your mentor if you prove ready to seek information as well as to request it.

Observing, questioning, interpreting and speculating

Earlier, we referred to the importance of questioning within clinical placements and noted that questions often have to be reserved until later. It is worth anticipating what that will feel like, so that you can ask questions more strategically when you are in the placement. Figure 6.1 outlines what typically happens.

1. Observations and experience

Learning starts with experience, and clinical placements provide a constant stream of experience. It is difficult to decide what to focus on, what to consciously observe and what to think about and what to let slip by. You cannot observe everything, neither can you analyse the whole experience before you. It is normal that you process only a percentage of the information available. Your observation will become more purposeful if you do four things.

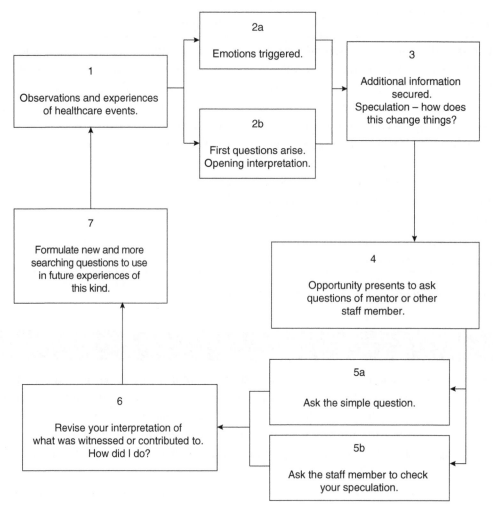

Figure 6.1: Learning in the clinical setting

- Note what seems most important to the patient. This usually means reading first and foremost what could entail risk for them and, after that, the events that may determine their experience of the quality of care. For example, the patient reports that they are allergic to penicillin. This needs noting down and reporting to others.

- Remember the learning outcomes that you need to achieve and the skills you wish to develop. It may help if you distil these into four or five priority interests. Lengthy lists of learning objectives are difficult to remember in the clinical area.

- Look for patterns of behaviour and sequences of events that seem to tell a story about the nature of nursing care. For example, patient admission to hospital is a storyline and one that involves several nursing skills.

- Relate those observations that interest you most to your previous teaching. Does this confirm what you learned in class? Does it modify your understanding or augment the information that you received there?

2. Questions and emotions

Two things happen simultaneously at this point. You will certainly experience a number of emotions associated with what you experience in practice. You might note excitement, admiration, encouragement, confusion, disappointment, cynicism or anxiety. Experience is 'in the raw' here and you are confronted with an insight into nursing that may or may not support your preconceptions. The goal here, then, is to acknowledge honest feelings but not to have them derail your learning. If you worry about, wonder at or even disapprove of something witnessed, allow for a moment that you might not yet have all the information to allow a full evaluation. Mentally save those feelings and formulate a question about them for later. For example, 'I noted that you were very firm with Mrs Brown's daughter this morning. She had been warned that her mother would be discharged this week. Does that approach work best?'

Alongside the first emotions will be some questions in your mind and some initial interpretations of what is going on. These will constitute your first ideas about what is happening. In the above example, you may have wondered, 'could the nurse have seemed more empathetic towards this relative?' or 'what is at stake here, rehabilitating the patient, freeing up a much needed bed or expecting of a relative a shared duty of care?' If you are alert, you will begin a tentative interpretation of the event: 'I suspect that this nurse has few choices. The need to attend to lots of patients places some limits on the extent to which she can personalise care.'

In the early stages of your course, you might notice a number of frustrations associated with nursing care and the organisation of services you meet during placement. Absolutist thinking (as summarised in Table 3.2 on pages 50–1) is characterised by set values and quick judgements. Something is right or it is wrong. It is good or it is bad. Care may be worthwhile or useless. It is extremely tempting to think in these ways while you are yet naive about the pragmatics of health care. While patient dignity and safety are critical in all circumstances, it is nonetheless true that care is often collectively managed in one institute or another. So priorities have to be identified and sometimes patients are supported with a holding care measure or explanation. It is well worth talking to your tutor about these emotional experiences, those relating to what you believe should happen and what seems more realistically to be the case. On the one extreme, you must of course be prepared to report malpractice but, on the other, you must manage a lifetime career in the profession where care prioritising is a skill in itself.

3. Additional information

It is likely that the stream of new information will continue coming your way. You need then to store your first thoughts and allow a new layer of thinking to develop. You are in the business of speculating. At this stage, there is no guarantee that your ideas are correct but speculation is still required. So, in our example, we may learn from the ward secretary that Mrs Brown's daughter works full time and that she has already lodged a request that her mother stay in hospital until the weekend. She was aware of the planned discharge but hoped to argue that she could support her mother better if she were available during her first days at home. The additional information probably demonstrates the daughter's concern to be an active carer but leaves doubts, too, about whether she trusts the other community care arrangements that have been put in place. You find yourself speculating further about systems and service, and about professional and lay care liaison. The nurse needs to work with a system but to advocate, where possible, the concerns of lay carers too.

4. Question opportunity

Opportunities to question arise later and in a variety of guises. It may be a one-to-one chat with the staff nurse during a coffee break or an opportunity for expression of concerns during a shift change. Nurses, doctors and others might invite questions after a ward round. The majority of such opportunities will be managed away from the audience of patients and lay carers. As we see below, there are two sorts of questions that could be asked but, irrespective of which you choose, it is necessary to demonstrate a respect for colleagues.

5. Asking your questions

Sometimes the complexity of things observed makes it difficult for you to pose anything other than a very simple question. 'What was problematic about the situation with Mrs Brown's daughter? I sensed a tension there.' Better by far, though, and with a trusted mentor, is to pose a question that invites them to check out your early speculation about events. 'I noticed the difficulty with Mrs Brown's daughter and started mulling over what that might be. I sensed that she wanted the discharge to work with her own arrangements; that she was really motivated to help with the transition home. But then again, she might have also been distrustful of the arrangements that we have made too. It isn't easy to find the compromise and we have to live with the discomforts of that … is that how you read it?'

6. Revising your interpretation

The answer you gain to your questions allow you to revise your interpretation of events. The interpretations may develop in several interesting ways and it is from this point that you can make some useful portfolio notes. For example, you might reinterpret your skill at reading practice episodes. Do I seem to be improving? You might re-examine your understanding of the mechanisms of hospital discharge and return to relevant policies.

7. Forming new questions

Having summed up your thoughts in the light of feedback, you are ready to observe practice with new insights. In our working example, you might consider in more detail how clinical colleagues work incrementally towards hospital discharge of a patient. How soon do they start preparing patients and carers for this? Do they always hear and understand what others are saying? In the end, are there economic and logistic tensions that inherently underlie such things?

Activity 6.3   *Critical thinking*

Study Figure 6.1 and consider whether the process of steps described there might assist you to be a more strategic learner in clinical practice. Why is it important to attend to what each step teaches us during the course of a placement?

Working with your mentor

Students are not always aware of what a mentor brings to clinical supervision, so let us start with that. Mentors are experienced practitioners, who are familiar with their area of care and its local policies and protocols, who have undertaken a short course in the principles of learning, teaching, support and assessment, and who are charged with guiding you during your clinical placement. They act as advocates of learning but they also have responsibilities to inculcate you into the team and its work (Price, 2012). They work assiduously to help you to master necessary skills and apply your knowledge, but retain responsibilities towards their patients, colleagues and the profession. Mentors share unique insights into practice wisdom – the practical ways of conducting nursing work (Price, 2013).

Successful work with your mentor will:

- help you to manage your anxieties about learning in the clinical setting;
- help you to develop an acceptable approach to enquiry in this setting;
- open doors to other expertise in the clinical setting (a mentor might introduce you to colleagues with specialist knowledge and highlight your enthusiasm as a student);
- give you thoughtful and honest weekly feedback, so that you are well prepared for assessments and end of placement reports;
- help you to address your own learning agenda as well as that required by the course.

Activity 6.4   *Communication*

Pause to think about how you can establish an early rapport with your mentor. Make a list of things that you could do and give a short rationale for each.

The working relationship with the mentor should be one of trust, purposeful work and mutual respect. Mentors expect students to arrive ready and eager to learn in the placement setting. Not all mentorship relationships are equally satisfying, however. It is possible that you will complete some placements where you feel that you did not achieve a good rapport with your mentor. You may still have passed the assessments and gained new insights, but it was much harder work than one where the mentor seemed enthusiastic, receptive to your enquiries and ready to gently challenge your assumptions. Search for, savour and celebrate the exceptional working relationships with mentors and acknowledge your own hard work with the less satisfying ones. Then ask some reflective questions. Could you have approached matters differently? Sometimes circumstances are against you both, for instance where staff sickness disrupts the continuity of your supervision.

As the working relationship develops, opportunities exist to deepen understanding between you and to begin to explore what it means to work as a nurse. Table 6.2 describes some of those opportunities and includes reflections from Gina on what does or does not seem to help.

Managing assessment

Reports are linked to clinical placements. They cover matters such as the development of your skills, the attitudes that you demonstrate in practice, your commitment to nursing care and the gains made in your knowledge there (Bennett and McGowan, 2014). In previous times,

Learning opportunity	Gina's notes
Evaluating your own performance, for example associated with a clinical procedure.	*It is a mentor's duty to give you honest feedback on your performance, but sometimes you get the best of this when you ask for their comments. You need to indicate that you're ready to hear constructive criticism.*
Sharing some doubts about your ability or understanding.	*You pay the mentor a compliment when you confide a doubt, and the best of them really appreciate this. I did so concerning my maths and the calculation of drugs. My reward was a series of mini teach-ins that boosted my confidence.*
Talking honestly about a team relationship that worries you.	*You won't get on with every member of the team. I think that it's good to try to resolve issues in the placement if possible. In one instance, the mentor was able to explain why a consultant seemed brusque and I felt reassured that I wasn't doing something wrong. Remember, though, you cannot expect the mentor to help you if the discussion remains completely secret. The mentor might need to represent your concerns elsewhere.*
Expressing some hopes and aspirations about future nursing work.	*I hadn't thought about this, but you're right! We need to keep dreaming. It helps us keep going when times seem tough. There were mentors who encouraged career aspirations.*
Securing recommended reading.	*Yes. I have even been loaned books and articles by a considerate mentor. But, remember, the library doesn't shut because you have gone on a placement.*
Celebrating your successes.	*The first person to congratulate me after I passed my first placement report was my mentor. It wasn't a perfect performance, but the mentor said to me, 'Do you realise how rare it is to achieve such warm comments from so many different professionals?'*
Appraising what needs to be done to meet objectives, to pass assessment.	*Definitely. The end report should never be a surprise and, if you're open with your mentor, you will get lots of warning about what needs improvement.*

Table 6.2: Mentorship-linked learning opportunities

assessment was formalised as a series of events and these events were linked to key tasks, such as the medicine round. Today, assessment is said to be 'continuous' and we need to consider the psychology of this process. The first thought that many students have is just how daunting it seems: 'During a clinical placement I am likely to make many mistakes, say a number of "wrong things" and inevitably alienate someone!'

There does need to be judgement on performance and this remains an issue for qualified nurses. Annual staff appraisals, complaints by patients and reviews by auditors are all part of professional life. Assessments that are made of your performance are mediated by an understanding of your stage of training and the learning objectives set; they comprise inputs from a number of staff members and take account of both the 'good days' and the 'bad days' of your time in placement (Price, 2012). The staff are interested in your learning and your response to guidance. While you might demonstrate shortfalls in skill or knowledge, these can often be compensated for by a willingness to receive instruction. What makes it very difficult for mentors and others to pass a student on their placement are shortfalls in skill and/or knowledge, combined with a refusal on the part of a student to change.

To help you to manage assessment, you need to be critical of your own performance and to search for gaps in your skill or knowledge. You will need to recognise misconceptions that are not serving you well. Such a personal audit of week-by-week performance will then enable you to seek the guidance of your mentor and, at the earliest possible point, to start correcting any short-falls and building on your successes. The following represent a series of week-by-week questions that might help you to evaluate your progress.

- What do you think was the best of my work this week and what still needed improvement? (Notice the search for both. It helps to receive praise as well as constructive criticism. Recognition of effort and attentiveness will stand you in good stead.)

- If you were to suggest one focus for improving my practice next week, what would it be and why? (Sometimes it is important to focus on a specific area and, if you can demonstrate a major improvement here, you will show your ability to reflect and develop.)

- How do you think it feels for a patient to be nursed by me? (This is a bold question, but patient experience is everything. An exploration of what represents quality there can be very useful.)

- I have written down three things that I think I am good at and three things where I think I could do better. Would you check whether I have made good choices? (Here you are using the 'check my speculation' approach, which is powerful because it shows your openness to change and reveals where you think there could be problems. At worst, the mentor will gently point out your misconceptions and you can refocus your efforts. At best, you are told honestly that you underestimate yourself in several regards.)

Assessments of your performance during a clinical placement will focus on your skills, the way in which you apply your knowledge and on your attitudes and values. The judgement of skills is usually well received by student nurses. They understand that the mentor, and others who contribute to the assessment of your performance, are themselves skilful. Receiving critique of your applied knowledge is also usually well received, at least, where the mentor and others have asked you pertinent questions. It seems fair to critique applied knowledge where you have had opportunity to reason aloud and to demonstrate why you think or proceed as you do. Assessment of attitudes and values however can sometimes be contentious and it often feels hurtful. This is because your attitudes and values are inferred by what you do, what you say and how you approach care and colleague relationships. When students struggle in this area of their learning, skilful coaching may need to follow in the next placement (Kelton, 2014).

Pause to reflect on how different the campus and the clinical environment are as places of learning. The robust enquiry and debate attitude that is so important on campus might seem aggressive in practice. Absolutist thinking, something that we have equated in Chapter 3 with lower levels of critical thinking and reflection, may in practice become stereotypes that have been applied to patients, relatives or professional colleagues. It is vital that nurses learn to explore and respect the concerns of others. If you label individuals ('she doesn't care about other patients, she thinks we're there just for her!') or groups ('trying to get doctors to listen to patients' worries is like drawing teeth'), this may indicate to assessors that you have not paused to consider all possible explanations of events encountered. Remember, transitional thinking is characterised by the consideration of different possibilities. We imagine that situations might not be as they first seem. This, at the absolute minimum, is what you should be aiming for.

One of the ways to demonstrate your positive attitudes and values relating to care is to seize opportunities to discuss care philosophy with your mentor and other senior staff. If you demonstrate an enquiring and respectful interest in what is being done, you are much more likely to convey favourable impressions to others. So, for example, you might reflect that a patient's struggles with alcohol addiction clearly make it harder for their liver to recover and that this distresses you too. You wish that patients could behave more rationally as regards using substances that carry risk. But then you acknowledge, too, that you have not really ever confronted addiction yourself. In expressing distress that the patient risks their health by excess intake of alcohol, you express compassion. In acknowledging that you do not understand addiction completely, you convey humility. Students are usually well evaluated where both compassion and humility are combined. To evaluate others as 'wrong', 'stupid', 'naive' is likely to convey an arrogant attitude.

Whatever you proclaim regarding your attitudes and values, though, remember that deeds speak at least as loud as words. Have you worn your uniform correctly? Have you been punctual? Have you shown a due degree of flexibility as regards what others need to do? Are you polite? How do others know that you are listening attentively to what they tell you, especially if it is something that seems unwelcome to you? The patterns of shifts that you complete as a student on placement are a foretaste of what work will feel like. For nurses to trust you as a colleague, they must feel sure that you will attend on time and work with interest in what the team is trying to achieve. Part of the contextual thinking that you learned about in Chapter 3 is associated with work and practice ethic, getting the job done in a professional, effective and efficient manner.

If you have received critical commentary as regards your attitudes or values, we recommend the following:

- Clarify what, specifically, the mentor is referring to, without challenging the assessment itself ('can you just help me with that point, I need to understand which colleagues I have seemed dismissive of?'). A mentor should be able to cite examples of where your behaviour has seemed problematic. Better still they can articulate the conditions under which this happened. Perhaps you seem more dismissive when under stress?

- Ask how the assessment was made. It is unusual for a mentor to reach this judgement by themselves, so ask whether they have conferred with others before reaching the judgement. A professional mentor will have conferred on such matters, realising how unsettling such an evaluation can seem. If the mentor relates how several different colleagues have noted the same problematic, it is highly unlikely this is simply a matter of opinion.

- Ask whether there was any counter behaviour which seemed especially good to offer a different impression of your attitudes and values. It is quite reasonable to ask for assurance that the balance of your behaviour has been considered too.

- Take the criticism away and think about it, before raising your concerns with the mentor or link tutor associated with the placement you are concluding. If you wish to raise points about these matters, write them down and acknowledge both strengths and weaknesses in your practice. Confronting mentors with the challenge 'you're all wrong' is unconvincing and suggests a lack of insight. It is better to explore a problem with the same humility and interest as you have been recommended here to approach the placement as a whole. A placement report may still record concerns about your attitudes and/or values, but these may be mediated too, by your willingness to explore behaviour afresh and identify some areas for improvement yourself.

Chapter summary

There are several key messages in this chapter. Learning in clinical practice is different, sometimes intense, and you must be an active and organised learner. You help shape the learning experience by working with your mentor and using the steps described in Figure 6.1. Learning in clinical practice need not seem chaotic, confusing or inaccessible if you think critically about what you encounter and continue to ask questions about what you experience and achieve. Part of your learning work is to accommodate the emotions that attend new experiences. Pausing to mull these over will enable you to ask sensible questions later on. It takes time to resolve emotional differences between what you think should be and what could be – between *my way* and *their way*.

A cycle of inquisitive questions will not by themselves guarantee learning. You will need to invite questions and challenges from others. You need to search out and carefully consider the feedback you receive. It can seem bruising to face a criticism about something you thought you were good at, but remember, contexts change and what worked in one place might not be appropriate in another. Nursing is a craft, an art and a profession that works within contexts. Mentors in particular do not give critical feedback lightly, mindful as they are of how vulnerable learners can feel. The feedback will usually be carefully considered and supported afterwards with a review of what might improve matters.

Forming a good working relationship with your mentor significantly increases your learning opportunities. In a trusting relationship there is scope to express doubts and to confront long-held fears. You may, like Gina, resolve a difficulty that liberates your learning throughout the rest of the course. Building a rapport with your mentor offers the prospect of a placement that not only teaches you a great deal, but provides you with a great deal of learning pleasure.

Further reading

Dinkin, S, Filner, B and Maxwell, L (2013) *The Exchange Strategy for Managing Conflict in Health Care.* Maidenhead: McGraw-Hill.

Clinical areas are sometimes places of conflict, those relating to values, resources and priorities. This textbook for conflict modellers and teachers offers much that can be used by students, mentors and link teachers as they review what seemed problematic as regards attitudes and values within the clinical arena.

Price, B (2012) Key principles in assessing students' practice-based learning. *Nursing Standard*, 26(49): 49–55.

This article explains just why the assessment of learning in practice is a sophisticated process and sets out principles for fair assessment of students.

Sharples, K (2011) *Successful Practice Learning for Nursing Students*, 2nd ed. Exeter: Learning Matters.

This volume provides further in-depth discussion of the process of learning within the clinical setting, and includes further material on working with a mentor and preparing for your placement.

Standing, M (2014) *Clinical Judgement and Decision Making for Nursing Students*, 2nd ed. London: Sage/Learning Matters.

This valuable book leads the reader through different ways of thinking about clinical decision making and explains how an understanding of ethics, reflection and priorities can lead to better decision making.

Walsh, D (2014) *The Nurse Mentor's Handbook: Supporting students in clinical practice*, 2nd ed. Maidenhead: Open University Press/McGraw-Hill.

This book includes clear indication of excellent mentor practice but also that which is less helpful. If you encounter difficulties working with a mentor it may be helpful to draw on the principles of best practice as you explain your worries to the mentor or link tutor.

Useful websites

www.nmc-uk.org/code

Nursing and Midwifery Council: The Code: Professional standards of practice and behaviour for nurses and midwives (revised 2015).

Studying the revised and updated version of the NMC Code is vital. This document responds to many of the criticisms of nursing care that have arisen as healthcare provision struggles to meet the demands of an ageing and a growing population. While there seem a lot of nuanced responsibilities to address, many are clustered together around due concern for the patient, their information, collegiate working with others and sustaining live updates in your learning as a professional.

www.cetl.org.uk/learning/tutorials.html

City University/Barts and The London Hospital School of Medicine and Dentistry, Centre for Excellence in Teaching and Learning.

One of the best ways to develop and revise clinical skills is to watch video recordings of excellent practice. Although clinical skills may be practised slightly differently from institution to institution, it is still helpful to explore resources such as these to better analyse what may seem problematic while learning in practice.

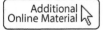 For examples of analytical essays and other useful material, please visit the companion website at **www.sagepub.co.uk/price_harrington**

Chapter 7
Making use of electronic media

NMC Standards for Pre-registration Nursing Education

Because the subject matter covered by electronic media varies widely, there are no specific standards to link to. The skills covered in this chapter underpin how you successfully learn and achieve all the standards, within the environment of electronic media.

Chapter aims

After reading this chapter, you will be able to:

- summarise the ways in which electronic media communication influences critical thinking;
- identify the ways in which electronic media might enhance the quality of your learning;
- explore personal feelings, aspirations and concerns regarding the use of electronic media within your course of studies;
- identify ways in which tutors provide feedback on assignments and how this could be used;
- prepare appropriate contributions to electronic forums associated with your course of studies.

Introduction

We have seen in earlier chapters how the environment in which we learn plays a role in shaping our thinking. In the clinical setting, for instance, the way in which we ask questions is influenced by the nature of the clinical work. In workshops, thinking is moulded by the exercises that we engage in. Learning to use the current electronic media is as much a part of successful learning as is command of a subject or practice skill. We need to realise what opportunities the media offer.

Electronic media are widely used within nursing courses to support student learning, networking and skills development. If you complete your studies at a distance, the part played by electronic media may be even greater. Email, electronic conference forums, wikis and electronic noticeboards and cafes have become a significant part of the course experience. You may, for example, get feedback on assignments by email and perhaps engage in debates online. Seminars might be conducted online or you might build a communal resource of information, something that the student group can all use (by means of a wiki, a place where students communally post information).

In this chapter, we examine what is involved in learning using different electronic media and make suggestions about how you can derive benefit from them. We acknowledge some of the anxieties associated with the use of these media and explore the ways in which they advance your ability to think critically. To illustrate critical thinking and reflection in action we refer to two case studies. The first of these is the handling of emailed assignment feedback. The second relates to electronic forums and concerns the development of arguments around best nursing practice.

Messages and the media

Just how important learning media are to nurse education can be illustrated with some items from an imaginary time capsule dug up from your garden. Within it, you find:

- a 1960s medical-surgical nursing textbook;
- a chalkboard and a set of chalks;
- an overhead projector and some acetates;
- a computer-based instruction program that teaches you the nursing process;
- a file containing discussions from an online course forum.

Activity 7.1   *Reflection*

Look at the above items and decide how you think each of these may have shaped the teaching and learning of nursing. More profoundly still, do you think that they also influence how we as nurses think and reflect?

During the 1960s and 1970s, medical-surgical nursing textbooks were a key resource in the training of nurses. Typically, the chapters were divided into accounts of illnesses, their treatment and then the associated nursing care. There was a lot of emphasis on nursing procedures and tasks, and it was accepted that nursing care was largely dictated by the treatment ordered by a doctor. Were you to read such a textbook today, you might remark how formulaic the care seemed. Nurses were instructed to think, but did so within carefully prescribed boundaries.

You may have already encountered teaching using a chalkboard or perhaps a whiteboard. What is significant about it, though, is the way it concentrates learning on the teacher. 'Chalk and talk' teaching involved the teacher lecturing an audience and periodically placing figures or lists of points on the board that the student was required to copy down. While students could be invited to use the chalk or whiteboard themselves, teaching was usually in one direction – from teacher to student.

Overhead projectors caused similar problems. Lessons were determined by what was prepared on the acetates that were placed on the machine projecting images on to a screen. The tutor could swap and/or re-order the sequence of acetates but the agenda for what was to be taught was largely pre-set. Scope remained open (as before) for conversation, but the breadth and depth of critical thinking and reflection were usually still constrained by the mindset of delivering the required content of the session. This same thinking, based on delivery of required information, was still influential in the early computer-based instruction programs. As a student, you would work through the series of on-screen pages, complete the simple tests that appeared periodically, and then finish the lesson, perhaps noting at the end your final score.

It is the file of the online forum discussions, however, that represents a significant departure in terms of learning and teaching. Depending on how the forum is run, there is scope here for students as well as tutors to set agendas, for students to lead sections of discussion, and for the whole to be based solidly upon discourse. While tutors may well have 'posted' (positioned) resources here (such as hyperlink connections to important library materials), and may have moderated the conversation in terms of acceptable contributions, the learning is strongly cen-tred on shared reasoning. The higher levels of critical reasoning and reflection that you read about in Chapter 3 are supported by just this sort of learning. While it is more active and harder work for students than listening passively to a lecture, it is also the sort of learning which helps you to explore your beliefs and values and to venture arguments that others will then test. If all the other items within the time capsule nurtured private learning, the online forum expected communal and arguably expansive learning (that is, learning that demonstrates the evolution of ideas, arguments and reflections, shared by other members of the group, and that remain on record in a way other forms of teaching often do not). It was necessary to think aloud.

Activity 7.2   *Reflection*

Having completed Activity 7.1, reflect on your feelings about the different learning styles that seem to be demanded in association with the media discussed above. Do you think of yourself as someone who is more comfortable learning privately or publically? Being honest about these reflections is important, because it influences what you take from electronic learning media within your course.

Today, an even wider selection of online learning activities might be encountered:

- reviewing or building web logs (blogs) of your own (accounts of professional life and practice, a form of open diary which requires careful thought if you are not to contravene university or code of professional practice rules);

- reviewing or making podcasts (short passages of information that may be presented in audio or video form);

- engaging in simulation exercises, where you control an avatar – a persona – within a case-study situation;

- building professional networks, perhaps international ones, using facilities such as Skype or Social Learn (**http://sociallearn.open.ac.uk/public**).

Email

Your use of electronic media (e.g., Facebook, Twitter, mail-order websites) in the past may have been linked to things such as social networking, online shopping and text messaging using a mobile phone. Students vary widely in their electronic media experience and older students may feel less electronic media 'savvy' than their younger peers. Upon joining your course, though, it is likely that you will be linked to a course webpage within the university and will have an email account set up for you so that you can communicate more flexibly with your tutor, the library and study group colleagues. Email extends the campus in significant ways. Through email, you may receive a 'study group message' from your tutor that is broadcast to the group as a whole. Using email, you might be encouraged to develop a 'study buddy' working relationship with one or more other students. Sometimes a more senior student is asked to mentor a more junior learner and email aids communication.

Just as there is etiquette associated with the use of electronic forums ('netiquette'), so there is one associated with the use of email for educational purposes. Beyond the usual caution that to type in CAPITALS is rude (it equates to shouting), there are other, equally important, rules associated with what is and is not to be discussed using an email. For example, you may discuss a draft piece of coursework with your tutor or personal tutor by email, but to do so with a study buddy might be to risk censure. This is because of the university rules concerning academic collusion and the need to ensure work is not plagiarised. It is wise, then, to check university rules associated with academic collaboration and to consider what this means for your use of emails while at university.

Wikis

You may not have encountered a wiki before joining your course, but it can simply be described as an electronic space where individuals make contributions that add to the understanding of a subject (Honey and Doherty, 2014). Individuals type their entry to the wiki in a text box, check what they have written and then post it to the wiki space on the course webpage. The purpose of a wiki is to add layers of information – extra interpretations of what has been posted as the subject of the wiki. So, for example, your tutor may have invited the study group to contribute examples and definitions of the term 'rehabilitation'. In this way, as each of you adds a small contribution (typically a paragraph or so), an extended definition of the concept emerges, which might later be discussed as part of a tutorial. The wiki remains online as a reference resource for you and others to draw on later.

It can seem strange to build a resource of this kind if you have been accustomed to thinking of knowledge as 'out there', something to be accessed within the library and beyond. You might wonder on what authority you and your colleagues have a right to create knowledge of your own. In truth, though, the world of healthcare knowledge is constantly recreated and adjusted by individuals. Nurses need to interpret existing knowledge drawn from elsewhere and to reinterpret it in the context of changing healthcare circumstances. They need to draw on their practice experience as well, because not all the important or best knowledge has been published. So wikis are very important. They help accustom you to actively creating or reconfiguring knowledge in ways that are pertinent to the requirements of professional practice today.

Activity 7.3   *Critical thinking*

Make a few notes on the following.

- What are the attractions and responsibilities associated with wikis?
- Are they useful as a means of helping you to develop your own reasoning?

Electronic forums

Most courses offer electronic forums, which are places where students and tutors can communicate with one another, either asynchronously (i.e., over time) or synchronously (i.e., at a designated time when all participants are asked to be online together, so communication is more immediate). As with wikis, you access the relevant electronic forum using your student identification number and individual password, a process that ensures the relative privacy of discussions within that space. At the informal end of the spectrum, electronic forums are designated 'cafes' and you are free to discuss a wide range of topics connected to university life. At the more formal end of the spectrum, individual forum discussions are connected to course modules and postings made there may demonstrate your 'attendance' or even contribute to course marks achieved.

In the formal forums, a series of individual discussions is initiated (often by the tutor) and, as each student adds responses of their own, a 'thread' develops. At different points the tutor may tidy up the thread, editing material so as to ensure the final record of discussion remains comprehensible to students. Also, in editing the thread, work is undertaken to ensure accessibility. It is not done to change your thoughts or points, save only where you post something that goes beyond what is allowed by the university as being respectful to others.

Electronic forums are, of course, rather different from the tutorials and related discussions you might share in a classroom. For one thing, a record exists of what each has contributed. It is possible to audit trail the discussions as they develop. This can seem a little worrying if you equate conversations here with records of performance. It takes a little while to appreciate the forums are places of honest and thoughtful speculation. Wise tutors assist with this by very clearly signalling which forums are used for assessment purposes and which will not feature in the evaluation of your progress.

Activity 7.4   *Communication*

- Given the above description of electronic forums and the posting of messages there, how does this form of communication differ from the conversations you share face to face?
- What are the advantages and the disadvantages of the different forms of communication, and how might they affect the way that you represent your thinking to others?

Electronic classrooms

Electronic forums are valuable, especially the asynchronous ones, as you have the opportunity to visit them when it suits you best and to leave contributions as and when you can. They wait for you to play your part. But nonetheless the conversations can seem a little slow or stilted. Threads of discussion can take a long time to develop, undermining your commitment to the communal learning work. For this reason, many universities are developing their own bespoke electronic classrooms or using commercially developed ones. One example of an electronic classroom is Elluminate (**www.elluminate.com**). Electronic classrooms are designed to function as tutorials within the online environment and they offer significant benefits when it comes to managing study time. There are no car-parking or public transport expenses associated with attending these tutorials, but you will need access to a modern computer that runs the latest software and have a head-set microphone so you can participate successfully.

You join the electronic classroom using a pre-set web address (a URL) and log in with your student password or number. What then appears is a whiteboard screen upon which you or your tutor will be able to draw diagrams, make lists or sketch flow charts. Beside the whiteboard screen there is a series of control features with which you need to acquaint yourself using the university training sessions. Commonly, these features include:

- a facility to ask questions or make points (using your microphone which must be switched to 'live' to work – remember to switch it off after speaking);

- the opportunity to vote in debates or in response to tutor questions (tutors often use this to check that you are all comfortable with the teaching so far);

- a facility to view streamed video or audio material, or to follow a PowerPoint presentation the tutor presents on the whiteboard screen;

- the opportunity to visit other web addresses using hyperlinks provided (highlighted words that take you to a new place if you click on these with your mouse);

- a facility to move to a 'breakout' room where you conduct discussions with a smaller group of students.

The use of electronic classrooms within nursing faculties is still comparatively new, and tutors and students are still exploring their potential. They usually require a little technical preparation (configuring your computer) and some discipline (especially in the use of microphones if others' work is not to be impeded). They can seem unfamiliar insofar as you do not necessarily see the faces of other students (as you might with a webcam-supported Skype discussion). Against that, however, they provide real-time, interactive learning for students who might not be studying on campus and may extend the support facilities you would otherwise enjoy at the university. Using an electronic classroom you develop computer-facilitated conferencing skills that may be important in your future healthcare work.

Making good use of feedback

We come now to the first of four case studies within this chapter and one designed to help you to make the best use of electronic media to develop your learning. As part of your coursework, it is possible that you will submit both formative assignments (those that are not awarded a grade) and summative assignments (those that do secure a grade) electronically to your tutor

> Children have particular difficulties expressing pain. Younger ones have a more limited vocabulary to describe the pain and may use general terms like 'tummy' to refer to its location. They don't have a clear sense of time and may struggle to describe the duration of the pain. MacGrath (1989)[McGrath (1990) in your reference list[ER1]] explains that nurses have to use parents to help interpret the pain. Parents are familiar with the way in which a child expresses themselves and can help determine whether pain may be a problem, for example when the child seems distracted and unable to concentrate on what they are doing[ER2]. Children have just as much pain as the rest of us and it's wrong to assume that they don't feel pain in the same way as adults[You need a reference here and perhaps to consider making this a separate paragraph. This paragraph is all about the expression of pain and your last point is about the incidence or nature of pain encountered].

Comment [ER1]: Are there more recent references that you could use?

Comment [ER2]: Do you think there are any circumstances when we need to be more cautious about relying upon a parent to help interpret a child's pain? If you are unsure, why not look up 'Munchausen by proxy' syndrome?

Figure 7.1: Examples of track change and margin note commentary feedback

and receive your feedback in a similarly paper-free way. Electronic submission has the advantage that you can obtain a record of the assignment being submitted on time. Also, you have more time to complete the work (you do not need to factor in time to mail hard-copy assignments or wait until a study day to hand them in). One of the other key advantages of an electronically submitted assignment is that the tutor can give you both summary feedback (as an end-of-work commentary) and feedback in the form of textual annotations that you can read as part of an attachment emailed back to you (see Figure 7.1).

Figure 7.1 illustrates two forms of feedback on a single paragraph extract from a student's assignment answer. The first is called 'track changes' and is presented here as underlined text that appears within the body of the essay work. In the first instance, track changes has been used to correct the presentation of a reference. The adjustment shows the correct spelling of the author name and queries the date of publication. In the second track change, the tutor provides guidance on both the referencing of the work and the planning of coherent paragraphs. Each paragraph should have a distinctive subject. The second form of feedback consists of marginal annotations using the 'comment' feature. ER in this instance stands for 'educational reviewer', although initials can be changed to reflect the name of the tutor. ER doesn't stand for 'error', because some margin annotations can be used to congratulate you on your work: 'Michelle, this is excellent, you summarise the theory with great skill!'

While the volume and complexity of written feedback on an assignment answer may vary, good feedback remains unambiguous. There are no unexplained ?s and !s dotted around that leave you to guess what the tutor means. The question then remains: what purpose is the feedback fulfilling, and how will you make sense of it and what will you do next?

The purpose of feedback

One purpose of feedback is to correct a misapprehension, whether it concerns a reference, a drug calculation or an assertion about ethical care. Corrections are often handled using track changes, with the tutor either deleting something and inserting the correct material, or commenting on the deficits. But other feedback may have a more subtle function. Comment ER1 in

Figure 7.1 is designed to prompt some further thought and enquiry. While this form of challenge is designed to help you to improve work, other challenges are more rhetorical and are designed to illustrate the way in which the tutor is 'thinking aloud' beside you (ER2). Tutors do not invariably expect you to respond to such remarks, but may leave them for further consideration. On occasions, the marginal commentary is intentionally provocative as well as rhetorical, as in this example: 'Perhaps we are naive to imagine any of us can completely assess the pain of another. Pain is bound up with private experiences, memories and fears. I wonder what you think?'

In these ways, the feedback you receive within a returned assignment becomes a delayed conversation. The tutor indicates, 'This is what I noticed, this is where I wish to guide you and here is where reflections could go a little further.' At best, feedback starts to model critical thinking for you, and reviews the state of current knowledge as well as your answer to a set question.

Making sense of feedback

We need, then, to make sense of the tutor's feedback. Does it require a response on my part? Does it prompt some new work for me? Am I invited to request some additional help? However important a coursework mark or grade might seem (and we note this first of all, don't we?), the commentary that accompanies your assignment answer is the most useful of all. Even if you have achieved a good mark, there is always something more to glean from the commentary provided. Why is this a good essay? Seeing the pass mark, noting the warm tone of the tutor's feedback and heaving a sigh of relief are not enough. You need to ascertain what the tutor thinks you have learned here and what could remain to be achieved.

Doing something with feedback

While, logistically, tutors supporting large student groups cannot enter into protracted dialogue with every student, there is a strong case for corresponding further with your tutor in the following circumstances:

- where you have secured a poor grade and where the commentary suggests you have misunderstood the question;
- where the commentary suggests a significant gap in your subject knowledge (that gap may prove important in later assessments);
- where the feedback has posed new questions to you (you wish to ask the tutor to help clarify a matter);
- where the tutor has suggested other possible lines of enquiry.

It is understandable to worry that you may inconvenience a busy tutor, but if they signal the above things, they really do welcome contact with you. At this point, you need conviction about the purpose of the assignment. Yes, it may be a test of your progress and may come with a grade, but it is also part of learning. The conversations that follow on from the assignment feedback will help you to develop your powers of discrimination and argument formation.

Reflect on any assignment feedback you have received to date and answer the following question.

- Did I use this to help develop my critical thinking/reflective practice?

If the answer is no, decide next why that was.

- Did the electronic form of communication put you off, making it seem impersonal?
- Or, on the contrary, did it make receiving feedback easier?
- What have you perhaps lost by not seizing this opportunity?

Making arguments in the forum

Our second case example of electronic media-mediated learning concerns the use of electronic forums. Tutors use these forums for various purposes, including the development of study group conversations (learning from one another), as a means of collecting together a range of views, and as a means of helping you to track changes in your collective thinking (tutors can archive forum discussions and later invite your group to examine changes in reasoning). Making contributions to the forum, and especially arguments online, can seem more difficult, though. We asked Fatima to complete Activity 7.4 (see page 111) and here are some of her reflections on contributing to forums:

I have enjoyed the different forums that we shared during the course so far. To read other people's ideas and to have them there, at midnight if you wished, is something that I never thought would be possible. But posting my ideas was more difficult. It was easy to support someone else, to say 'yes I agree' but more difficult to make a case, to suggest something of my own. I found myself thinking, 'this is not polite, to insist in this way to my colleagues'. My personal tutor smiled and noted that in my clinical placement I was described as 'a bit quiet'. She was right, I have not been brought up to assert myself and I know that nurses must do that. But there is a difference between class and computer. In class I can say things. I make my views heard. In the computer, though, the words last forever; they are there on screen and, just as I can read other people's words, so they can read mine. I feel exposed by that and worry that, if my words seem unwise, I will suffer.

Fatima's reflections are familiar to tutors. As another student once put it, 'Debating in the forum is like making a maiden speech in Parliament. An audience is listening to you and it will be recorded.' However, making arguments is necessary if you are to advance your thinking. There is a need to formulate arguments and to test them with supportive peers and an empathetic tutor. Happily, the system for posting forum messages involves composition and there is a chance to review your posting before it is electronically submitted. While most students do this to check their grammar and syntax (worrying about presentation), the greatest benefit of the pre-submission check is being able to consider whether your points seem coherent and clear. No one in the forum expects perfection, especially in a synchronous discussion, where postings happen a little faster. No one anticipates that their comments will always be supported either. Just as in other conversations, there will be some good points made and some that seem more questionable. Making a clear argument, though, is something that we can practise when we edit messages before they are posted.

Activity 7.6   *Critical thinking*

Imagine that you are engaged in a forum discussion about the right (or otherwise) of individuals to end their own lives. The last posting made by another student (Susan) expresses a deeply held religious conviction that patients should not exercise such a right and that, to do so, relieves healthcare practitioners of the responsibility to search for and deliver quality-of-life support measures. Now it is your turn to offer something. Consider the three short arguments below and decide which, if any, you might post to the forum. We discuss the merits of each below but encourage you to evaluate them first, as this will help you consider how to prepare postings to forums. Whether you support one or any of these postings will depend in part on whether you are clear on your views concerning end-of-life decisions.

1. I can see Susan's point regarding who should have the right to curtail a life, but it is fair to observe that significant numbers of people do not express a religious conviction and question whether there is an absolute law here. We might need to remember other healthcare philosophy that we operate with. Perhaps there is a link to consumerism. If we require patients to make choices in other areas, for instance as regards medication, why are they not capable of making such decisions about death?
2. One of the things that we wrestle with is how patients' decisions make us feel. Their actions seem to reflect on us. 'I ended my life because you couldn't help me.' This seems a terrible thing and yet these are views we can imagine patients holding. In another year, they might have other choices available to them.
3. The media debate concerning this topic is often about the intentions of those who facilitate death. If there are inheritance benefits being sought, or if the death of the person simply makes life more convenient for others, ending a life undermines all that is dignified in society. If the decision is truthfully about the relief of suffering, and acknowledges that quality of life has gone, perhaps we have to support carers.

We would start by stating that this is a very powerful debate and one that would only be undertaken by confident students. It is not a place where a new student would be expected to start. The formulation of an argument here, however, is shaped by:

- concerns about what you think and wish to convey (being genuine about your own beliefs);
- issues concerning how this will seem to others (audience reaction);
- clarity of what you wish to convey (easy or difficult);
- whether you wish to make a new point or contest a previous one;
- coherence (can I demonstrate a reasoned point?).

Response (1) above gently contests the point made by Susan, noting that it is the beliefs of the individual patient, as much as those of the practitioner, that should help determine how end-of-life decisions are made. The point is well reasoned. If patients have responsibilities as healthcare consumers, they also have rights. The argument could be developed further, but it is clear. If we were making this argument, though, we might end with an invitation that shows that we are posting in speculative mode: 'Does anyone else hold views on this? I'm just searching through this idea about how being a consumer affects things here.' What is important is that the argument made needs to be measured and open to speculation by others, otherwise the point made could seem bigoted. The person posting this argument feels comfortable that they are expressing an authentic position (one that highlights individuality), and that their point is coherent (if patients have responsibilities as consumers, they should have rights too).

Response (2) seems tangential to the point made regarding religious convictions and end-of-life decisions. It acknowledges our discomforts about such decisions and illuminates the problem, without necessarily expressing the student's position. It might express an 'I simply don't know' perspective. Your position does not instantly have to be shared in the first posting – it could be something that you edge towards through discussion. There is nothing wrong with such contributions to a forum, as they offer extra dimensions to think about. Later, the tutor may sum up these considerations and pose some new questions.

Response (3) seems to move on to a new area of argument – that of consequences and carers. What if relatives or friends help someone to die? The link to the current point about rights is there, but not as directly as we might expect. Had you made this argument, it would certainly still be welcomed as thoughtful and reflective. Later, though, it might be moved to another discussion – one associated with how we should see the role of the lay carer. What is important here is that new points should be targeted towards the discussion topic. It is harder for others to make use of your argument if it wanders elsewhere.

What can we say, then, about the business of making arguments within electronic forums? First, it seems necessary to accept that forums are not the same sorts of conversations that we share elsewhere. While they are collegiate, they are not transient. They leave a record and it is for this reason that you will naturally wish to compose your arguments carefully. Second, successful forums are permissive and allow that ideas and arguments will develop within and through them. You will make several postings and the clarity of matters will improve as the group takes stock of what has been posted. It is OK to 'feel your way' in these matters. Your tutor has a key role here, helping to sum up points. Third, discussions held there are not and should not be reputation busters. Your tutor should make this clear at the outset, otherwise trust will not grow within the study group. Provided basic etiquette guidelines are followed, the forum remains a place for speculation and the practising of arguments.

You are likely to enrich your critical thinking by recognising the multiple perspectives that exist on a subject within the forum. Your views will not necessarily be those of others and the tutor does not relieve you of this uncertainty by stating that 'nursing has this view'. You will develop your reasoning ability because you have to formulate points that others can understand and relate to. Notice, for example, the connection made to consumerism in response (1) above. This student reminds companions that, if we subscribe to a consumerist philosophy, we cannot so easily abandon the free-choice principle in the matter of end-of-life decisions. It may take practice to represent such points, drawing on your observations and experience, but the effort that you put in here may well pay dividends later in writing assignment answers.

Interacting successfully within the electronic classroom

In the third case study, we turn to successful learning within the electronic classroom environment. Although you have already learned valuable principles while reading about learning from lectures and seminars, there are some subtle variations here that you need to be aware of. Much of what you need to consider now relates to attending sensitively to the needs of fellow learners and making the technology work for everyone. As you cannot see other class participants, you have to imagine how they feel as they interface with the classroom using a computer.

We start with strategy. Your strategy should begin before the class itself and should ensure that you are well prepared to play an empathetic and inquisitive role during the session. Preparation begins by noting on what date and at what time the class session begins. It can be very disruptive to join the class late and then try to catch up on what has already been done. To ensure that you can contribute fully, it is necessary to do a brief computer check. Most of the electronic classroom platforms have a log-on wizard facility that allows you to check that you can hear the audio output clearly and test that your microphone is working well. Running these sound checks well in advance of the class should ensure there is much less chance you will undermine others' learning because of a technical difficulty. Familiarise yourself with the various control functions at your command within the electronic classroom. In advance of the class, check to see that you can turn your microphone on and off (the screen icon will change, usually with the microphone raised when it is live and facing downwards when it is off). You need to have your microphone off when you are not speaking as otherwise your open channel microphone might block a fellow student.

The classroom is likely to have a separate box where you can type in text, a question, a reflection or a request. Conduct a trial run before the class to ensure that your typed text appears in the box as expected. Your tutor will be able to see this while running the session. Do not assume, however, that all such typed text responses are instantly acted on. Responses to such student feedback may be saved for a summing-up point. Identify whether you are able to indicate your understanding of the session using emoticons (smiling or frowning faces). Your tutor might rely on these to determine the pace and the direction that the class takes.

The final check is to understand what form the class will take. Will the tutor allocate the first section of the class to a presentation, in which case will you be asked to offer questions at the end or during the session, perhaps using the typed text box? Will the class constitute a workshop, in which case the first section consists of tutor instructions on what you are asked to do? If it is the latter and you work within a breakout room, at what time are you meant to rejoin the class? The running of an electronic class needs to be more formally planned than one on campus, so if the tutor has not already spelled out how you will proceed, do not be afraid to ask in advance of the class or at the start of it.

Attending to the class itself requires a little extra thought as well. Remember, you will be seated before a computer screen, possibly many miles from the university itself. The tutor cannot readily see if you are listening intently or whether you look interested or bored. So we recommend:

- that you ensure that your chair is comfortable and you can easily use the keyboard, without stretching (classes typically last no more than an hour, but can still make demands on you, so a good posture/position is important);
- that you have a notebook and pencil to hand (you may wish to compose queries or reflections carefully before posting these within the electronic classroom);
- that you have refreshments to hand (avoid spilling liquids on the computer, however);
- that you use the 'out of the room' icon to indicate when you are not present in class (otherwise it can be frustrating for the tutor and fellow students, who might wonder whether you have been lost to the session because of a technical fault).

Class sizes vary, but a key consideration is to post responses, either typed or audio, that seem constructive and that do not dominate the discussion. Remember, you cannot see the scowls of other students in this environment. So monitor whether others have already typed in questions or reflections within the text box and, where possible, save your points for the frequent, 'are you all happy?' breaks that experienced tutors tend to use. If you wish to refer to something specifically, note down the location in your notebook: 'I have a query about slide 4 in the PowerPoint presentation ...'; 'I'd like to reflect on the third whiteboard diagram, this seemed important because ...'.

Where students agree, classroom sessions are often archived; that is, they are recorded, so that you and colleagues can access them again later. If this has not been agreed, however, you will need to make notes as you proceed through the class. Larger presentations, for instance PowerPoint, are often transferred to you by the tutor, so you can download them on to your computer for later reference. Anticipate, however, that at the end of the session you may be asked to conclude what you understood, and what you have taken from the class. Having notes to hand will help you to do that and to indicate what you hope to follow up study on. As with face-to-face lectures, the notes made here are likely to be brief and will need expansion after the class has finished.

Because you cannot readily see one another in the electronic classroom, it is necessary to be very well organised in any breakout sessions. Determine quickly who will be the 'chair' of this discussion and who will be the secretary – making notes that can be fed back to others at the end. If you were the chair during the last breakout session class, suggest a new colleague for that role now. Volunteer to act as secretary if you have not done this recently; working purposefully and quickly together is a key part of what makes electronic classes successful.

Activity 7.7   *Communication*

Make brief notes about circumstances under which you think an electronic class might be especially helpful for you and other students. Note the queries that you have regarding getting the most from each session. Alerting your tutor to your worries and interests in advance of classes may mean that the session is arranged in a new way, one that helps you derive the maximum benefit. If you already know who will be fellow members of a breakout discussion group, contact others in advance to agree who will chair and who will act as secretary for the forthcoming session.

Evaluating website information

The final case study within this chapter concerns the critical evaluation of website information. Quite commonly within electronic learning, you will be invited to conduct a search on the internet and will then be asked to critically examine what you found there. Chapter 8 provides additional guidance on the critical examination of evidence but we also need to add some remarks on the internet as a source of knowledge. The internet represents a new frontier of information, much of it unregulated and some of it arguably spurious (Haigh and Costa, 2013; Roberts, 2010). While the internet can be liberating, it can be misguiding as well.

The internet comprises service providers who offer the search facilities using addresses (URLs) or search terms, website providers who provide the home for internet content, and content authors. In many instances, the website providers will be the content authors as well. So, for example, if you go to the website for the Nursing and Midwifery Council (**www.nmc-uk.org**) the content provided will be authored by the Council itself or its approved researchers or consultants. In other instances, however, a website may provide facility for different authors to post their content. The website owners note that the content found there does not necessarily reflect their views. The website is acting as a conduit for debate and opinion. One of the strengths of the internet is that it provides a forum for a wide range of views and insights, some of them cutting edge and of the moment. There is a minimum of regulation, save for that demanded by governments to protect the vulnerable and to maintain standards of decency or limit criminal activity. The internet remains a contested space. There are always agencies who seek to regulate it more and those who insist that it is a place of free speech.

One of the first questions that you should pose when you find internet information, then, is who are the authors? Who makes the claims presented here? In many instances, there are no authors named in website information; the conventions of published books or articles do not apply. It is then necessary to examine what they argue (searching for possible bias) and to determine whether the authors' perspectives may have been shaped by the owner of the website. For example, you find a paper on the part played by sugar in the human diet and this makes a number of assertions about why it is beneficial. Arguments about the possible contribution of sugar to a greater incidence of obesity are given little or no attention. The paper is found on the website of an organisation with close associations with several processed food manufacturers. Caution may then be required and you might question whether the information found is impartial. You might ask the question, would this website allow publication of material that ran counter to its commercial interests?

A further important question to ask regarding internet information is when was it published? Whereas in providing a reference for your own work you will indicate the date when the website was accessed, the issue remains, are you clear how old the information found is? The best papers included within websites have both author details (and their professional or employment affiliations) and details about when the paper was uploaded to the website. Many others, however, will lack one or more of these details and then you will need to be circumspect about whether you can recommend this resource within your review. If the information was integral to the website itself (rather than an embedded paper) you might check the last date that the website was updated. This is sometimes stated within the 'home' page. Even then, however, a recent update of the website does not necessarily assure you that the material that interests you has been critically re-examined. Updates are conducted for a variety of reasons and the latest one might not have concentrated on what interests you.

Activity 7.8 — *Research and evidence-based practice*

Choose a subject to research on the internet – so much the better if this relates to a controversial subject, such as the causes of obesity, the rights of a particular patient group, cigarette smoking or similar.

Use the facilities of your internet service provider to identify relevant websites and choose one of these to scrutinise in greater depth. How easy was it to ascertain who authored the website information, and what affiliations they had, especially that which is 'front of shop', rather than any papers that are included there as resources? Check whether the information provided seems to support the stated position or mission of the website owners (often expressed as 'our mission' or information 'about us'). Check to see whether the website provides information about when the site was last updated and against what criteria.

In examining websites as possible sources of information, the appropriate attitude is one of healthy scepticism (Guardiola-Wanden-Berghe et al., 2011). It is not necessarily the case that the information found is not valuable but, without details of its origin, what it indicates may be something more about the website and its mission than about work reported. In health care, as elsewhere, commercial, ideological and political influences may play a role in shaping what is provided. As a critical consumer of this information you will need to ask questions about what interest the information might serve – whether it was provided for your needs or those of others.

Chapter summary

In this chapter we began with the argument that communication media have an important influence on the messages shared, and we hope that we have proved this point. The way you reason using electronic media will be different from reasoning in class. This is not to suggest, however, that these media in some way undermine the critical thinking and reflection that can operate here. The quality of feedback possible with an electronically submitted assignment, the excitement that can be generated in an electronic classroom, the richness of information on the internet and the depth of debate possible within an electronic forum can be exceptional. The very fact that you can access conversations at times to suit you, and that there is space to compose your answers with care that is not available in a real-time face-to-face conversation, highlights the critical thinking opportunities here. Electronic media make a major contribution to 'thinking time'; they prompt you to reflect before you speak and this is valuable. At best, learning within the electronic media expands your horizons and helps to develop your enquiry skills. The internet offers a multitude of information, some of it of excellent quality.

continued ... •

Electronic media are not without their challenges, and you may have observed through the activities within this chapter just how different this communication can seem. For some, it feels artificial, especially if students are private and contemplative in nature. If electronic learning environments are used without clear thought, as an unimaginative substitute for face-to-face activity, the reputation of electronic learning quickly deteriorates. It is at its best where the tutor marshals fascinating resources to which the class has prompt access, that then form the focus of attention for discussion. Tutors are becoming adept in creating welcoming and supportive electronic learning environments. They recognise the anxieties that can lurk as you prepare your first postings, and they know that to contribute to something that remains 'on record' undermines the confidence of some. Acknowledging these concerns, they arrange feedback and summarise discussions in ways that demonstrate tolerance, an appreciation of your efforts and a commitment to imaginative new ways to learn.

Further reading

Ford, N (2012) *The Essential Guide to Using the Web for Research.* London: Sage.

Ford's book is a step-by-step guide to locating and using information, sourced on the web, within coursework you complete. The web offers huge potential in terms of the variety and richness of information available, making this a very valuable guide.

Health and Care Professions Council (2014) *Professionalism in Healthcare Professionals: Research report.* London: HCPC. Available to download at: www.hpc-uk.org/assets/documents/10003771Professionalism-inhealthcareprofessionals.pdf

One of the best ways of conducting a seminar is to base it on a new piece of research or a professional body report. This one is a very good source example; it explores the way professionalism (and its limits) is understood by a range of healthcare professionals regulated by the Council. Nurses have their own code of conduct, but it is instructive to understand professionalism as it is thought of by others.

Hutchfield, K (2010) *Information Skills for Nursing Students.* Exeter: Learning Matters.

For those interested in extending their information skills by using the internet this is a welcome volume. There is clear guidance on searching for information and managing that which has been gleaned. The text is written in clear and accessible language.

Wheeler, S (2015) *Learning with E's: Educational theory and practice in the digital age.* Carmarthen: Crown House Publishing.

Steve Wheeler is a long-time observer of electronic learning and an active blogger on the subject. His textbook provides an interesting overview of e-learning in its widest sense, how it influences notions of learning and teaching and what this might mean for society when e-learning is the norm rather than the innovation.

Useful websites

www.lib.vt.edu/instruct/evaluate

Virginia Tech Libraries Service: Evaluating internet information

Most university library services produce some sort of guide to evaluating web-based information (we suggest you check yours), but this one is well laid out and covers in a simple aide memoire table the questions you should be asking of internet information found.

https://kb.wisc.edu

University of Wisconsin (Learn@UW Knowledge Base)

It is easy to be naive about what it takes to develop and run a successful online discussion group. This university guide reviews what is required and highlights the importance of types and volume of inputs that should be required of students. In counterbalance it is emphasised that tutors must structure and manage the conversations in an active way so the learning seems purposeful.

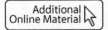

Additional
Online Material

For examples of analytical essays and other useful material, please visit the companion website at **www.sagepub.co.uk/price_harrington**

Part 3
Expressing critical thought and reflection

Chapter 8
Critiquing evidence-based literature

....

NMC Standards for Pre-registration Nursing Education

This chapter addresses the following competencies.

Domain 1: Professional values
All nurses must act first and foremost to care for and safeguard the public. They must practise autonomously and be responsible and accountable for safe, compassionate, person-centred, evidence-based nursing that respects and maintains dignity and human rights. They must show professionalism and integrity and work within recognised professional, ethical and legal frameworks. They must work in partnership with other health and social care professionals and agencies, service users, their carers and families in all settings, including the community, ensuring that decisions about care are shared.

9. All nurses must appreciate the value of evidence in practice, be able to understand and appraise research, apply relevant theory and research findings to their work, and identify areas for further investigation.

Domain 3: Nursing practice and decision making
All nurses must practise autonomously, compassionately, skilfully and safely, and must maintain dignity and promote health and wellbeing. They must assess and meet the full range of essential physical and mental health needs of people of all ages who come into their care. Where necessary they must be able to provide safe and effective immediate care to all people prior to accessing or referring to specialist services irrespective of their field of practice. All nurses must also meet more complex and coexisting needs for people in their own nursing field of practice, in any setting including hospital, community and at home. All practice should be informed by the best available evidence and comply with local and national guidelines. Decision making must be shared with service users, carers and families and informed by critical analysis of a full range of possible interventions, including the use of up-to-date technology. All nurses must also understand how behaviour, culture, socioeconomic and other factors, in the care environment and its location, can affect health, illness, health outcomes and public health priorities and take this into account in planning and delivering care.

....

continued ... •

1. All nurses must use up-to-date knowledge and evidence to assess, plan, deliver and evaluate care, communicate findings, influence change and promote health and best practice. They must make person-centred, evidence-based judgements and decisions, in partnership with others involved in the care process, to ensure high quality care. They must be able to recognise when the complexity of clinical decisions requires specialist knowledge and expertise, and consult or refer accordingly.

Chapter aims

After reading this chapter, you will be able to:

- outline the different ways in which evidence might be defined;
- referring to paradigms, summarise why evidence needs to be critically analysed in different ways;
- discuss validity, reliability, transferability and authenticity as key criteria by which to examine evidence;
- use insights from the debates about knowledge to explain why, although evidence-based practice might be desirable, it may also be difficult to achieve.

Introduction

During the last decades of the twentieth century and the opening decade of the twenty-first, there has been an exponential growth in the volume and complexity of healthcare evidence (Moule and Goodman, 2014). Evidence, in its different guises, has become a key source of knowledge for nurses and the need to think critically about evidence has grown as a result (Scott and McSherry, 2009). Nursing leaders urge their colleagues to ensure that practice is as evidence-based as possible. This has obvious advantages for the patient (where incontrovertible evidence supports one or other intervention) and for the nurse, who otherwise faces a quandary about what represents the best practice. Because there are many different things that the nurse could do, and because there are different arguments about what the nurse should do, all nurses need to be very sure of evidence as a support for their practice. Much may be gained through the judicious use of evidence, but responsibilities remain too. All nurses need to evaluate evidence in a clear and well-reasoned way.

To explore this subject, we return to the four students we first met in Chapter 1. Each has searched for and begun to engage with evidence within the healthcare literature. But as we shall see below, critical thinking, when it is applied to evidence, is not straightforward. Evidence is neither a neutral nor a straightforward concept and the way in which evidence is defined may influence how it is then evaluated.

Activity 8.1	*Critical thinking*

Below we set out the opening definitions of evidence that Stewart, Fatima, Raymet and Gina have used to search for information. We asked them to enquire about pain and its management. As you can see, they are quite different and, as a result, different sorts of literature were subsequently found. Different sorts of evidence critique will need to be used.

Decide which of the student definitions of evidence seem most convincing to you. Prepare arguments for your colleagues as to why this particular definition seems appropriate.

Case study: Four definitions of 'evidence'

Gina: 'I've always thought of evidence as that which science and in particular experimental research or randomised controlled trials produce. What distinguishes evidence from mere information is that the knowledge has been secured by design; there is a rigorous method to the work and we can evaluate that. So, for me, there is an emphasis on pain interventions, medication and other treatments that might make a discernible difference.'

Fatima: 'May be! But you're missing something here – evidence isn't restricted to research. Audits, patient satisfaction surveys, case studies of unusual patient situations and needs, what we did to look after them, that counts as evidence too! Pain is individual and sometimes circumstantial, so we need a wide-ranging appreciation of it.'

Raymet: 'So what about the evidence of your own eyes, then? If reflection doesn't produce a sort of evidence too, aren't we missing out on something? Not everything can be examined in a piece of research. Nurses accumulate insights into pain, the emotional as well as the physical sort, and that needs to be considered and reported on.'

Stewart: 'Perhaps, then, evidence is that which you can measure, that which you can quantify. Other sorts of information are still important but we shouldn't try to make evidence stretch so far, to serve every situation. We need evidence and patient stories – their narratives about coping with pain. Evidence, though – that should be apolitical shouldn't it? It should be produced by those who don't have a particular axe to grind about healthcare and how care should be!'

It might not surprise you to learn that evidence has been defined in all of the above ways, from either something quite discrete and distinct from other classes of knowledge to something that embraces a wide range of experience and insight (Gabby and Le May, 2011). Here, we suggest that evidence might be considered to be information that for the individual, group or organisation has greater authority than some other forms of knowledge, but which still requires scrutiny before it can be appropriately used. Information is contested, not only in terms of its authority but also whether it counts as evidence in the first place. To use evidence well, nurses are confronted with two profound and necessarily philosophical questions.

- What is the role of science in nursing? As science produces particular forms of knowledge, that which is described as evidence, should it underpin everything we do?

- If science is not to underpin everything within nursing, what are its proper limits? (Other forms of knowledge – philosophical, ethical, aesthetic, vocational – may have a role to play.)

Questions such as these cannot be evaded. Nurses have to acknowledge what premises they start from, and answering these questions lifts your reasoning into higher levels of critical thinking (see Figure 3.1, page 45). Is acceptable evidence universal or is it always modified in some way by a particular environment? Do our beliefs and values necessarily shape how we conceive of evidence and how we then approach the business of conducting research or our reviews of others' research? The discussion of evidence remains a discussion about philosophy, as well as about methods, data and results.

Debates about what represents best, appropriate or robust evidence are not always solely about judging how the evidence has been secured. They are sometimes about what knowledge nurses should use, and what should be the proper study and the basis of nursing practice. John Paley, for example, shows how philosophy and research design are intimately linked, shaping the sort of information that results and limiting, in part, its possible application in practice (Paley, 2014). If we research human experiences (that of the patient) then we may produce evidence that can tell us things about how nursing might be experienced, but we might not be able to predict outcomes for large groups of patients.

When the world-famous Cochrane database was set up (**www.cochrane.org/cochrane-reviews**), it focused firmly upon a quite discrete form of evidence, concerned with interventions and with cause-and-effect relationships. It focused upon treatments and what might be proven to work. Subsequently, the Cochrane database has considered a rather more wide-ranging collection of evidence, which relates to experiences in health care as well and which has been presented in the form of qualitative rather than quantitative data. It has been accepted that evidence in health care needs to relate to different things, not only interventions, but analysis of experiences, problems, perceptions and preferences as well. The need to diversify the understanding of 'evidence' has grown as nurses and others have become increasingly concerned with healthcare quality, and quality has been understood in experiential as well as effectiveness terms (Ransom et al., 2008).

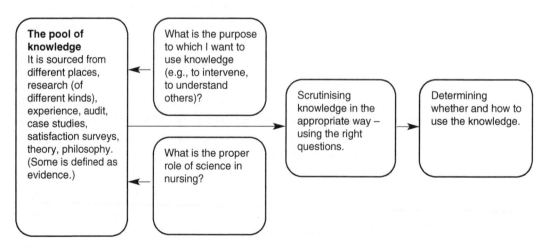

Figure 8.1: Approaching knowledge

Ellis (2013a, b) writes accessibly about both evidence-based practice and research but, here, the above students' debate has a particular critical thinking significance. We argue that evidence can only be critically evaluated when (a) the original premises of the research or other knowledge are understood, and (b) we understand the conventions for critiquing that particular sort of evidence. We need to understand something about knowledge and how this is conceived (ontology) and how that knowledge can be discovered (epistemology). You need to consider what your own attitude towards knowledge is, what is considered least and most important, and what you support as an essential resource upon which to draw when advancing nursing care (see Figure 8.1). Understand these things clearly and the critique of evidence becomes a more scholarly affair.

Knowledge and how to know it

In 2012, Thomas Kuhn's classic 1962 book *The Structure of Scientific Revolutions*, one of the most influential philosophy texts of the last century, was reissued. Kuhn was eager to explain that science did not necessarily evolve in an orderly sequence as knowledge and insights accumulated but that, periodically, there could be quite sudden and sometimes violent shifts in thinking and in what was accepted as truth. What represented incontrovertible evidence was, as it were, 'up for grabs'. Up until this time, science had seemed an orderly procession of ideas and had a clear function, which tended to focus on the manipulation of the material world, that which enabled human beings to order their physical environment in ways that were deemed beneficial. This period was called the modernist era (Rolfe, 2006), a time of rational endeavour where science was readily separated from other sorts of enquiry and reasoning, such as philosophy. A paradigm (a widely accepted conception of science, enquiry and reasoning) existed in association with the modernist era – one that today is called *positivist*. The positivist paradigm centres upon the empirical world, that which can be manipulated and tested, and can be controlled, or at least managed, within laboratory and (to a lesser degree) clinical settings. The positivist paradigm drew heavily upon research methods associated with the natural sciences, and work concentrated on trying to demonstrate and measure cause-and-effect relationships, the limiting of researcher bias and the testing of hypotheses (prediction of what would, or would not, be the case). Positivist science is classically associated with three things: accurate mapping, precise measurement and strategic manipulation (Bunniss and Kelly, 2010). Well-designed positivist surveys map or measure phenomena (e.g., anxiety traits within a group of patients) while experiments or quasi-experimental designs, randomised clinical control trials, manipulate things (e.g., use of new drugs to produce a therapeutic effect).

Activity 8.2   *Reflection*

Pause at this stage to reflect upon the implications of the positivist conception of research for nursing. If scientific knowledge comprises what can be manipulated under controlled conditions, how well does this relate to nursing practice? Are there conditions that you as a nurse can control within your practice, so that you can ascertain what impact a particular intervention had? You might think here perhaps of wound care, or perhaps the impact of breathing exercises as a means to help patients control anxiety and reduce their pulse rates.

The problem for many social scientists and nurses during the middle decades of the twentieth century was that the positivist paradigm, and its conception of science and knowledge, paid little attention to the practical conditions under which many people lived. The need to design studies that controlled for all undue influences (variables) meant that experiments could be exacting, but they might not relate coherently to practical care situations. Within the healthcare world, there was little chance of controlling all the factors that could influence how individuals behaved and, in any case, it was argued that people did not behave according to trait but (in many instances) according to circumstance. Predicting human behaviour was problematic. As a result of this, a new paradigm or collective world view began to develop, and to compete with the positivist paradigm. This new world view is sometimes referred to as the 'naturalistic paradigm', because researchers worked in social world conditions with fewer checks and controls on enquiry. The new thinkers were concerned that positivist science was too far removed from everyday life and that it was then difficult to use the results of research conducted there. Thinkers in the new paradigm admired work carried out by social scientists rather than those working in the natural sciences. The new paradigm is also sometimes referred to as the 'interpretive paradigm' because there was a greater freedom for the researcher to interpret data, especially experiences of others. But whatever we choose to call this new paradigm, it certainly includes a much increased concern with insights into human existence (Plested, 2014). There, phenomenologists explored the ways in which people made sense of their lives (Earle, 2010), ethnographers explored how common values and culture operated (e.g. Martin, 2015) and grounded theorists developed explanations of social processes (e.g. McCarthy et al., 2015). The work of the researcher was much less about designing tests and more about enquiring within the social world in an authentic and sensitive fashion.

Activity 8.3   *Critical thinking*

What do you think are the implications of naturalistic paradigm reasoning for nursing and nursing research? For example, researchers working in this paradigm are very concerned to reveal the different ways in which patients experience healthcare services and the support of the nurse (e.g., Little, 2012). But, because the researcher is less concerned with controlling the data, eradicating bias, the evidence resulting from this sort of research is often illustrative – it suggests what could be the case and expects the reader to determine whether their own experience matches what was reported. Recommendations, if they result from this sort of research, are much less prescriptive.

Today, researchers and philosophers of both paradigms work in what has been described as the postmodernist era (Rolfe, 2006), a time when there is much greater uncertainty as regards what represents truth and different explanations, and claims compete for the attention of practitioners. The matter is still more complicated, however, by the emergence of a third competing paradigm that also produces research. The *critical theory paradigm* was founded upon the premise that knowledge is rarely apolitical, that it is not neutral (Weaver and Olson, 2006). Instead, knowledge inherently carries power and there are many people within the world who are eager to deploy it to their own advantage. Marxist researchers (who challenge class or other political elites and their influence over the division of resources, including health care) and feminist research-ers (who argue that women and other disadvantaged groups are poorly served in health care and beyond) work within this paradigm. These researchers propose that investigators use research to expose injustices and to empower others to take greater charge of their lives (Freeborn and Knafl, 2014). As a result, a lot of research in this paradigm has been described as action research, consisting of cycles of collaborative activity to improve the lot of disadvantaged groups in health care (e.g., Kilbride et al., 2011).

Activity 8.4   *Critical thinking*

What are your reactions to this sort of science, where researchers are engaged in openly political terms, righting perceived wrongs or else empowering others to change the health-care world? This is research that is far removed from the positivist paradigm's concerns about bias. On the contrary, the researchers might argue that honest confrontation of ine-quality is the required starting point. Research exists to counter bias and injustice in health care. If you accept work from this paradigm, it has profound implications for nursing – how you use the research. You might engage in a polemical discourse – a series of arguments that are in favour of changing healthcare in particular ways.

Having formulated your reflections on critical theory paradigm research, turn back now to Chapter 3 and Table 3.1 (pages 48–9). There you will see described different levels of reasoning. Absolutist reasoning associated with research paradigms might be to conclude that there is only one sort of 'proper research'. You might fiercely argue this against all comers. But are there any advantages in linking paradigms of research to different contexts and care requirements?

As you think about the different paradigms, it might be tempting to conclude that you should take a particular stance: that which Gina argues is clearly right because …; Raymet's objections are appropriate because … But to back oneself into a philosophical corner might not prove that helpful. Nurses have to work pragmatically and imaginatively with different sorts of knowl-edge and a range of evidence within health care. It is, then, arguably appropriate to adopt a 'horses for courses' attitude towards knowledge underpinning nursing. Instead of arguing that one sort of knowledge is superior, that there is a justifiable hierarchy of better and worse evi-dence, it may be appropriate to venture that the key consideration is to what purpose is the evidence put. If we are currently concerned with an intervention and what works, it is likely we will search for and evaluate knowledge from the positivist paradigm. We will use questions that are appropriate there, which work with the claims of the research (research design and rigour). If we are currently concerned with insights, understanding patients or others better, we might search for information from the naturalistic paradigm and might ask different questions again. If a convincing case has been made for change, and the improvement involves a shift in power or opportunity, we might draw on research from the critical theory paradigm, and perhaps engage in research ourselves as part of an action research group. The key point is that we think critically in different ways and to strategic purpose. There is no one-size-fits-all way of reasoning possible here.

Asking different questions of evidence

It would be extremely helpful if authors of research evidence and other sorts of paper within the literature confided, at the outset, the paradigm within which they have framed their work. In practice, though, this rarely happens. Authors working within the positivist paradigm rarely allude to science philosophy supporting their work but move straight to the design of the survey or the experiment. It might be assumed from the outset by them that this *is* what constitutes science. They seem unaware of the wider philosophical debates about the nature of knowledge and how it is best known. Researchers working within the naturalistic and the critical theory paradigms are likely to be more explicit about their philosophical premises and may refer to a research approach that is clearly aligned to certain beliefs about the nature of knowledge and its role in health care. You get a clearer steer as regards the basis on which they are presenting data and findings to you.

Activity 8.5   *Group working*

To help you to test out our assertions above, arrange with colleagues to each secure a research paper on an agreed theme, perhaps pain and its management or similar (something of common interest to you all). Next, read your chosen paper, highlighting any passages of work that you think indicate the paradigm within which the work was conceived. Clues may be a focus on empirical data, traits, measurement, experimentation, and very detailed control measures in the research design, within positivist research. There may be reference to avoiding researcher bias – but be careful here – researchers working in other paradigms sometimes misunderstand bias and think that they must counter it in similar ways to researchers working within the positivist paradigm. Clues to research conducted within the naturalistic paradigm include reference to research approaches used there, phenomenology, grounded theory, much ethnography and, quite frequently, case-study research. There is an emphasis on natural working environments, on discovery and on insights into the experience of others. Clues to research conducted within the critical theory paradigm are terms such as *feminist* or *Marxist research*, and perhaps the use of *action research* – work designed to produce rather than investigate change.

Next, each summarise your paper to colleagues and then discuss which paradigm you think it originated from and what that might mean for its contribution to nursing practice. As some papers will probably seem ambiguous, identify those to your tutor and speculate where you think they *might* come from.

Questions in the positivist paradigm

Where it is concluded that evidence has been produced within the positivist paradigm, a group of questions become important (Furberg and Furberg, 2007). The first of these relates to the design of the research, and whether it has set out a clear question or hypothesis (a statement regarding what will be the case or will not be the case – the latter is referred to as a *null hypothesis*). The research has to be clearly structured and needs to state precisely which population of people it relates to and what the sample is. The way in which the sample was selected is important in this paradigm because, unless the researcher works with a whole-population sample, the sample is argued to represent the population as a whole. The reader has to be convinced that the sample constitutes a reasonable proportion of the population concerned and matches its key features (e.g., age distribution, gender, health circumstances, educational attainment). Statistical guidance is usually sought as regards what represents an adequate sample and, beyond that, a satisfactory return rate for questionnaires if a survey is used. Consideration of the population and sample size, the make-up of the sample and whether it is representative of the population affect study *validity*. The research is valid if it addresses the research intention set and attends to the sorts of situations and people that can relate to that. But small and unrepresentative samples of people can all undermine the validity of the research. They may report quirky data, which does not capture what the study population thinks or does.

A second concern within positivist paradigm research is *reliability* (Ellis, 2013b) – whether, using the same data-gathering methods and the same research design, similar results could be obtained at a later date. Of course, when dealing with human beings reliability could prove a problem. Positivist paradigm research works well where individuals behave or comment according to trait (those who see the world and behave in habitual and consistent ways) but it is less successful, less reliable, if people changed their attitudes, values, beliefs and behaviour on a regular basis – that is, behaving according to state (the situation prevailing). If people changed their mind frequently and behaved very inconsistently, it would be difficult to judge whether the research was reliable.

We asked Stewart to summarise why positivist paradigm researchers were so interested in things like validity and reliability. This is what he quite reasonably said:

> Well, the research is about judging something isn't it and if you're going to claim that something is or is not proven, then you have to be sure that all your methods are well organised, that the work focuses on exactly the right thing. You have to be sure that others could repeat your work, to check that they got similar results. Big decisions might rest on this sort of research, whether or not to use a particular drug, whether to start a new form of treatment. So the evidence needs to seem very robust indeed.

A further legitimate question regarding positivist paradigm research is that of bias. Has the researcher in some way, wittingly or otherwise, shaped the evidence so that it is not representative of reality (e.g., by using leading questions)? In positivist paradigm research a single and testable reality is assumed, one that can be measured and manipulated; that is, it is empirical. Has the researcher allowed others to shape the evidence in some way (failing to identify something else that affects an experiment but which has not been controlled for)? Positivist paradigm researchers are keen to control for bias and to limit the risk that rogue variables in some way shape the data in ways that undermine subsequent claims about it. It is assumed that in some sense undue influences spoil the validity of the data, so steps are taken to counteract this.

Controlling bias is a relevant concern in positivist paradigm research, which makes claims about empirical facts: 'This drug caused these reactions and we controlled for other possible influences by doing these things within the experiment'; 'This survey found out these things about this group of patients and the results weren't influenced by me using questions that only produced one sort of answer'. The researcher is concerned with the precision of the research – that it measures or manipulates what is intended and nothing else.

We checked with Stewart again, asking why he would be scrutinising positivist research for bias. He said, quite correctly:

> *Well I might put it this way. As the research is probably claiming something about the factual world, what is happening and will happen again and again, I'd want to know that claims made there weren't the result of some odd influence in the research, something that the researcher introduced because of his prejudices, or perhaps because of pressure from those who funded the research. So I would want to know that the recommendations that he reached about some new drug were indeed the result of the research and not who was sponsoring him!*

Questions in the naturalistic paradigm

The critical questions to be asked of evidence stemming from the naturalistic paradigm are different and much more about comparing the researcher's account against your own experience of phenomena. This is because the world is conceived of in less empirical terms. Everyone interprets their experiences and creates their own reality – their own account of what is really happening. So, for example, five people may visit the dentist and have treatment, but the experience and the meaning of these visits will depend as much on their perceptions of dentistry, dentists and what is likely to happen as the number of fillings they have. The emphasis here is on the perceptual world, that which is negotiated and even co-created (think, for example, about the meaning of old age: this is more than a physiological change (something empirical); it is a complex, interpreted experience). Because the research typically focuses upon experiences, perceptions and interpretations, and a multiplicity of these, it is important to examine how the researcher produced his or her account of phenomena.

Researchers working in this paradigm are not claiming to present empirical facts, a demonstrable truth that can be tested again and again, but a representation of what they have seen, heard and interpreted. Typically, the researcher deals with field observations and open-question interview responses, necessitating interpretation and the development of possible themes, and that which might convey what has been experienced. The researcher deals in the world of perceptions, interpreted by the individual who contributes to the research and then again by the researcher who cannot avoid using his or her own experiences to help make sense of what was said or witnessed. Because researchers are working with interpretations, it is accepted that what the researcher produces is at least in part a construction. So the concern with bias (so central in positivist paradigm research) is inappropriate. It is acknowledged that the researcher cannot but interpret and influence matters, for example through the line of questions that he or she pursues. Instead, typically, the researcher claims not to have controlled for bias, but invites the reader through a clear account of how the research proceeded (the audit trail) to determine whether what is reported seems authentic. In effect, the question is: in your experience has this sort of thing happened, have these sorts of concerns been expressed, or have these sorts of positions been taken? To illustrate, a researcher exploring perceptions of visits to the dentist first collects the narratives of individuals who have been through this experience. The research interviews have not been rigidly constrained by set questions and the researcher makes it clear to the reader that the questions within the interview were informed by his or her own impressions of what the respondent was saying. This may also have been informed by what past respondents have said. Researchers follow lines of enquiry, those that help to clarify their opening ideas gleaned from past interviews, or perhaps field observations. In explaining this (the audit trail), the researcher asks the reader to determine whether the research findings still seem trustworthy and valuable, as they return to the experience in question themselves.

Remember that, here, the concern is with insight and understanding of a phenomenon, and not with predicting what will happen in the future. So the first question you should consider asking is whether or not there is a clear audit trail that describes how data were collected and analysed. Was this by interview or by observation and in what order? How were the themes reported in the research arrived at? While all researchers need to describe the research design and steps taken, audit trailing is especially critical in this paradigm. This is because the researcher presents their own 'take on reality'. They provide their interpretation of what was heard or seen. As there is no appeal to an empirical truth, an absolute right or wrong interpretation, the reviewer of the researcher has to check the researcher's account of findings against their own experience of the phenomena. This is helped when the researcher shares how they arrived at their conclusions, especially as regards the data analysis process (e.g., identification of themes that help explain what was investigated).

We tested this idea out with Raymet, asking her about audit trailing and why this was important in naturalistic paradigm research:

> *I think it's because researchers here accept that a lot of the important things that nurses are interested in cannot be proven, they cannot easily be measured and predicted. After all, being ill is extremely personal. The disease might be empirical, measurable, but illness is an experience. Because of that the researcher has to access the patient's experiences and that does mean that they have to use a mix of questions, they need to find ways to relate to the patient. So when I come to judge this research I want to know about how they did that. I can then say, given this account and my personal experience of illness in the past this does or it doesn't sound convincing.*

As Raymet suggests, as well as asking questions about the audit trail, whether it was clear how the researchers proceeded, you need to ask a question too about authenticity (Green and Thorogood, 2004). 'Given what I already know about this phenomenon, do these findings seem credible?' The reviewer is asked to consider whether the findings 'ring true'. Of course, experiences elsewhere might not accord with your personal experience. They might be quite unique to another group of patients or practitioners. But, if the research evidence is to be transferable, if it is to be used locally, this concern with authentic, recognisable (but still possibly surprising and insightful) experience remains important. It is evidence that you can not only recognise, but might be able to do something with. Quite a lot of naturalistic paradigm, qualitative data evidence falters at this point. Human experience is contextual; it operates within a given context, a particular healthcare system (e.g., insurance-based health care, health care delivered in another culture where families care for patients in hospital). It may be authentic to local context but it might not be transferable.

Authenticity is subtly different from validity, because there is no assumption here that experience is empirical, that it remains constant and can be found again. On the contrary, human experience is dynamic, negotiated and changing, so data can never be definitive, only more or less authentic.

Questions in the critical theory paradigm

As critical theory research is polemical, consciously political, the first question to ask here is, are the researchers' premises about the need, problem or opportunity set out at the start? What is the research meant to correct or achieve? Honest critical theory paradigm research acknowledges from the outset what has framed and directed the research or what drives the researcher. The critical theory researcher would point out that truth is always contested, that the definition of what is happening is fought over. So every position is in some sense biased or partial, and reality is defined in terms favourable to a group holding power. But they concede a responsibility to set out their alternative truth, what concerns or alarms them, what they wish to correct or challenge. Having ascertained the researchers' premises and assumptions are clear, the critical analysis of evidence moves to an audit trail as above. How was the research conducted? Were the procedures here conducted in accord with the stated purpose of the research and the values of the researchers?

We discussed *action research*, a common method used within critical theory research, with Gina. She had seen action research under way in a clinic where she had recently been on practice placement. The research was all about developing a more consultative clinic, one that facilitated screening of sexually transmitted infections and contacts that the patient may have had. The researchers had stated that they felt the practitioners there were disempowered, being set targets and standards for tracing of contacts, but with little help given on how to create an atmosphere more conducive to screening and tracing work. The researchers negotiated a series of activities, first to help the staff examine their concerns and needs, and the training that they might require. A second round of activity explored with them their values and attitudes towards risk and patient needs. Patients sought a degree of privacy but the staff too needed to minimise risk for others, so work centred on facilitating responsibility in the patient. Gina observed:

> It was egalitarian research; it did attend to staff needs and concerns, but it didn't lose sight of responsibility too. Staff did have a duty of care to individual patients and they did have a public health responsibility too. So in that sense what the researchers did held true to their stated values and goals without alienating the managers who had set targets in the first place. It was about how to work better, how to be adequately resourced for what others asked you to do.

The nature of evidence-based practice

The discussion above illustrates why research evidence is by no means a simple thing; it comes in many different forms and has been conceived of in different ways. You will need to reason at a high level (see Table 3.1, pages 48–9) to do justice to a discussion of different sorts of research evidence. The purpose of research may be quite different, depending on how the research was conceived and where the information came from. For example, much research evidence within the naturalistic paradigm has been gathered to facilitate reflection. It raises questions such as 'Have you thought about this?'; 'Does this happen where you work?'; 'What concerns or needs haven't we attended to here?' Evidence associated with the positivist paradigm may contest current treatment or care; it might suggest what else works better, and the implicit questions are, then, 'Should we do something different?'; 'Should we continue doing this now?'

Evidence associated with the critical theory paradigm relates specifically to attitudes and values, the agendas and beliefs that might shape health care. Now the implicit questions are, 'Do you still believe in this?'; 'Are you doing something you truly value and can support?' Accepting the complexity of this, the different questions finally posed suggest that evidence-based practice will not be a simple or a one-size-fits-all thing either. The evidence-based practice may consist of changed care, because a critical mass of what works, and knowledge about what is safe and critical to the improvement in the patient's condition, has accrued.

Evidence from the positivist paradigm is drawn upon, and especially where that also accommodates consideration of the costs of health care. But evidence-based practice might also involve different ways to conceive of care partnerships, ways of working that show greater sensitivity to the needs of others. Evidence from the naturalistic or critical theory paradigm might be important here. Improvement in nursing care is still the central concern, but it is associated with different things, such as sensitivity, attuning care to patient requirement.

Successful evidence-based practice is, then, that which works with the strengths of different sorts of evidence, provided in association with different paradigms. Apart from nurse researchers, nurses do not usually 'make' evidence, that which is designed to prompt reflection or to illustrate experience, work as proof of what must be done. They suggest what could be done, given these insights. There is recognition of the limitations of evidence, and what may be claimed about it. Nurses and other practitioners realise evidence still requires interpretation and decisions about where and how best to use it. Evidence cannot substitute for clinical judgement and critical thinking. They need to be combined with these and to strategic purpose.

Fundamental challenges usually remain.

- Have we got enough evidence?
- Does it all point in the same direction and suggest broadly the same things?
- Have we got a mix of evidence, which attends to the aspects of care, what works, what is safe, what reassures the patient?
- Is the evidence usable; that is, does it seem to recognise the organisational, ethical, cost or political constraints and opportunities within which nursing operates?

Activity 8.6   *Critical thinking*

As you conclude your reading of this chapter, imagine that you are having a conversation with a friend who is thinking of enrolling on a nursing course. Your friend is very enthusiastic about the evidence that is now available to help patients. You are encouraged by her enthusiasm, but wish to ensure that she does not see evidence-based practice naively.

Summarise why the care of a chosen patient with a named condition probably needs different sorts of evidence and why each needs to be evaluated differently. Describe why evidence-based practice for such patients takes time to develop.

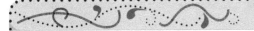

Chapter summary

You have now reached the end of Chapter 8 and your exploration of a particular sort of critical thinking, that which applies to evidence. While there are many other applications of critical thinking, especially with regard to the business of learning (see Part 2 of this book), the application of critical thinking to evidence is an overarching one. Evidence is one of the key knowledge bases on which nurses draw. It is extremely important and yet hotly contested. If you are to critically examine evidence, it is necessary to understand what sorts of evidence there are, how these are related to paradigms of knowledge and which questions are appropriate to employ there.

In this chapter, you have explored different conceptions of evidence and, while you have determined what counts as evidence for you, there may have been the discovery too that others see evidence very differently indeed. You might meet colleagues in the clinical area with different perspectives on evidence. To make sense of these sometimes fiercely argued discussions on evidence, you have looked at three paradigms, each of which shapes the ways in which people think about knowledge and conceive of evidence. Colleagues may or may not be aware they see evidence from a paradigm perspective.

The paradigms studied suggest a number of relevant questions to ask of evidence, those that are reasoned and respect what the researcher was trying to do. Using the right questions to interrogate evidence will help you to develop more reasoned arguments. You ask questions that seem relevant and help you to evaluate the evidence found.

Further reading

Bourgeault, I, Dingwall, R and De Vries, R (2013) *The Sage Handbook of Qualitative Methods in Health Research.* London: Sage.

Naturalistic and critical theory paradigm research has often been called collectively the 'qualitative' paradigm because of the types of data typically collected. This collection of edited papers provides a rich description of the varieties of research undertaken and the purpose of such research, and is an excellent resource.

Ellis, P (2013) *Evidence-Based Practice in Nursing,* 2nd ed. London: Sage/Learning Matters.

Peter Ellis provides a concise and highly accessible review of evidence-based practice and the important critical thinking that is necessary here. The book covers not only issues relating to the review of evidence but also the implementation of this within practice.

Harvey, G and Kitson, A (2015) *Implementing Evidence-Based Practice in Healthcare: A facilitation guide.* Abingdon: Routledge.

Having appreciated just how complex research and its evidence can be, you might reasonably wonder next how it can best be implemented? Different sorts of evidence might require different handling. This book explores exactly these issues and what facilitators have to do if they are to promote a more evidence-based form of health care.

Useful websites

http://consumers.cochrane.org

The Cochrane Consumer Network is an offshoot of the original Cochrane Collaboration (see below) and is designed to help members of the general public become involved in the evaluation of healthcare evidence and the systematic reviews that the Collaboration publishes. There is interesting video footage of consumers' views on this subject and guidance on how members of the public can access research evidence, working through the complex terminology there. The site is worth visiting because it highlights how others need to use critical thinking with regard to research and illustrates what can be done to facilitate that.

www.cochrane.org/Cochrane-reviews

The Cochrane Collaboration provides an extensive collection of systematic reviews of research evidence and a free to access handbook on how to plan these, ensuring a rigorous evaluation process. Systematic reviews are rigorous methodological interrogations of intervention research that are usually associated with what effects an intervention has. The Cochrane database provides an excellent summary of what has been evaluated so far. You could spend several profitable hours here, sensing just how critical the questioning must be before researchers' claims regarding evidence are accepted.

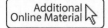

For examples of analytical essays and other useful material, please visit the companion website at **www.sagepub.co.uk/price_harrington**

Chapter 9
Writing the analytical essay

··
⟳ ᨒ ᨒ⸱⸱⸱⸱⸱ **NMC Standards for Pre-registration Nursing Education**

Because the subject matter covered in analytical essays varies widely, there are no specific standards to link to. The skills covered in this chapter underpin how you successfully learn and achieve all the standards, within the context of analytical essay writing.
··

Chapter aims

After reading this chapter, you will be able to:

- determine clearly the purpose of the analytical essays you are asked to write;
- identify the cases presented by others or the one you will deliberate on;
- adopt a clear position on the case within your analytical essay;
- select relevant evidence and link this to arguments within your written work;
- demonstrate more speculative and scholarly ways of writing in your essays;
- prepare conclusions that both sum up previous text and demonstrate what you deduce from it.

Introduction

During the course of your studies you will write a series of analytical essays, some of which you will tackle under examination conditions. No one assumes that what you achieve in examinations will necessarily be as good as what is managed within coursework. Without prior notification of the topics to be covered, you will write to best possible effect using your memory and any permitted notes. Time constraints limit your ability to plan, so you will need to use the precepts of critical thinking that you were introduced to in Chapter 1 and remember the basic structure of an answer, as explored in Chapter 3. Remember that, even here, it is important for your work to seem considered. There is little room for absolutist thinking, where you advocate only one cause, where you neglect the options, opinions and debates that encircle modern nursing practice. You will need to write in a more critical way even here.

This chapter combines our previous teaching on critical thinking and writing, and applies it to analytical essays. We remind you of some of the characteristics of more critical thinking that you first met in Figure 3.1 (page 45), and we direct you to example passages of higher level critical writing within the associated website resource (**www.sagepub.co.uk/price_harrington**). We consider the purposes to which the analytical essay is put and highlight the importance of establishing clarity of thought, and your position, before you start writing. We review how best to discriminate what should be included in the essay, and then the use of arguments that demonstrate your ability to weigh the merits and limitations of a case. We revisit how best to sum up the essay within the conclusion and make the point that success here consists of much more than simply repeating what has been presented earlier in the paper.

To help you to examine these points in some depth, and to see how a reasoned analytical essay looks, an example analytical essay (kindly supplied by Stewart, one of the four students associated with this book) has been made available on the website. Stewart's essay is not perfect, neither is it intended to become a template for exactly how you should write, but you can learn much from it. The work focuses on one subject – a review of how nurses make use of different sorts of evidence. It enables us to discuss analytical writing in the context of a specific question. At the point at which this essay was written, Stewart was nearing the end of his course. You should not assume this is a standard to be achieved from the outset of study. Read it, therefore, with a view to identifying what it can teach you about technique, and not as a comparison with your own work.

The purpose of analytical essays

Analytical essays are set for different purposes. The first of these is to test your understanding of a given subject and your ability to make a series of well-informed judgements about it (the evaluative essay). Such essays are frequently set as a review of the literature, research reports or healthcare policies. Examiners wish to understand whether you have a clear grasp of what others have argued, and whether you have developed a clear perspective of your own. Evaluative essays are sometimes set early on within a course to check your grasp of key concepts and ideas. If you do not understand these concepts, you may find subsequent learning more difficult and it will be hard for teachers to build on your raft of existing knowledge. So essays not only assess your knowledge, they tell the teacher something important about your reasoning process so far.

The second purpose of the analytical essay is to move forward from this, to assess your strategic thinking: what would you do next and why? These sorts of essays are frequently presented in the form of patient case studies, and here you would combine the declarative, procedural, knowledge and decision-making components of critical thinking discussed in Chapter 1 (the strategic essay). Classically, strategic essays of different kinds feature in the middle part of a course and they are set when the teachers believe that you have already amassed a variety of information that can and should now be applied to practice situations.

The third purpose is to test your ability to confront conundrums or to examine professional ethos (the philosophical essay). Essays of these kind often test your highest level reasoning skills (see Table 3.1, pages 48–9), because you have to ruminate on values and attitudes, priorities and principles in a way that shows you are thinking about care as a whole (that is, in metacognition). Sometimes, there is no obviously right or straightforward answer, and no neat solution, and the nurse has to manage a situation as it is. Papers about ethical dilemmas may be of this kind.

A command of care philosophy and ethics is important if you are to cope with the stresses of healthcare practice. Examiners want to know that you grasp the complexity of issues and the processes that will help you deal with these issues.

Activity 9.1   *Critical thinking*

Below are some essay assignment questions or instructions. Decide which purpose each of these questions serves. Visit the website resource (**www.sagepub.co.uk/price_harrington**) to acquaint yourself with Stewart's analytical essay and to determine which purpose this is meant to fulfil.

1. The attached case study describes the experiences of Avril, a 35-year-old woman with learning difficulties. She lives within a community home with five other residents. Read the account of Avril's relationship with Tony, another resident, and then critically discuss the challenges that arise in association with contraception here.
2. Nurses are necessarily interpreters of healthcare policies. With reference to a policy of your own choosing, critically discuss whether you support this statement. Remember to back up your points with reference to the literature and/or observations from practice.
3. As part of a new initiative to engage the public in strategic healthcare planning, four ex-patients have become consultants to your nursing team. How will you work with them to enhance the services delivered to patients? Make sure that you refer to theories of leadership and change agency taught during your course.

Our answers to this activity are given at the end of the chapter.

The case and the position taken

Having established the purpose of the forthcoming essay (what the question asks), our next job is to determine what position we take and what case will be considered. The two are not necessarily the same. A case might be stated as part of the question and you are asked to examine it. Question 2 in Activity 9.1 does that; the case is stated briefly, simply, that nurses are interpreters of healthcare policies. You present questions and arguments that explain your position on this given case. In other instances, you make the opening case in the essay and back this up with arguments. Under examination conditions, being clear about the case and position is critical. However, we are often so keen to make best use of the time available that we set to, writing down points that are confused. We seem unsure about the case and indecisive about our position. Yet we know that, by the end of the essay, our position has to be very clear. For example, relating to Activity 9.1, we might decide that we support the statement in (2) about nurses interpreting policy but with certain caveats. There are some restrictions, because nurses must simultaneously apply several policies and each demands priority attention. So, you might support the case that nurses interpret policy, but your position is a qualified one. It is vital then, before you write, even in an examination, to pause and consider what your position will be. If you have the chance to make a case of your own, what will that be?

Activity 9.2   *Reflection*

Stewart confided to us that he did not always clarify his position before writing essays. Certainly, his early exam work was 'position-confused', unlike the essay shared on the website resource. This was because he was fearful that the position he took would not seem the right one. He feared that examiners might judge him negatively if *his* perspective did not mirror theirs. He 'fudged matters', trying to write an answer that he hoped might please the examiner.

Reflect now on whether this worry has affected you too. Is it as important a problem as not knowing what your position is in the first place? Once you have done this, look back to Table 3.1 (pages 48–9) to remind yourself that, in academic settings, the last thing that assessors expect is that you will present an absolutist case, one that does not consider other possibilities. There is often no single right answer, only ones that have a clearer reasoning audit trail within them.

Establishing your position is important. This is because it will determine what arguments you make within the essay and what evidence you draw on. Some positions require a great deal of evidence to support them, reflecting the complexity and ambiguities of nursing care. If we continue with the above example, we would need to identify circumstances where:

- we definitely should interpret the chosen policy;
- there is more limited scope to interpret the policy;
- factors combine to severely restrict our ability to interpret the policy.

On balance, if we support the case, the first group of these factors should predominate. Showing that other factors intervene, though, and that there are caveats to consider, demonstrates that our judgement is not rash. In an essay such as this, we might draw on evidence from the literature that is connected to local protocols and standard care pathways, as well as observations from practice and discussions with colleagues who have managed policy implementation in the past. Explore our web page (**www.sagepub.co.uk/price_harrington**) to see different levels of academic writing (paragraph excerpts) which show the student setting out their position at the start of an essay and which help to distinguish different levels of reasoning that you met with in Table 3.1. We have purposively included weaker examples of writing to show the difference but, of course, you should aspire to more sophisticated writing wherever possible. Our notes explain what is stronger or weaker in the work presented.

Activity 9.3   *Critical thinking*

What sort of brief answer plan might you use in an examination situation to help you prepare an answer that demonstrates your position clearly in response to a question? Jot down an idea or two, perhaps describing a plan that you use now.

Our suggested plan is given at the end of the chapter.

Arguments and evidence

We have already seen in Chapter 3 that an essay is composed of a series of sections (introduction, main text, conclusion), which are, in turn, made up of a sequence of paragraphs, within which we advance our arguments. Coherent essays have arguments that fit with the position being defended and they lead appropriately to the conclusion. We might arrange the essay in several ways; for example, reviewing the alternative positions that might be adopted with regard to nurses' interpretation of healthcare policy, before revealing the position that evidence seems to support. Alternatively, our position may seem so strong that we state this at the outset, and then lead the reader through step-wise arguments that demonstrate its power. A committed stance of this kind is not simply absolutist thinking. The case is backed up by a series of carefully considered arguments in support of it. Some evidence is adopted and other evidence is challenged as being unclear, poorly articulated or perhaps less relevant to the context in hand. The assessor is left in no doubt that you have pondered your answer with care and taken the time to find and marshal evidence that supports it.

It is disempowering to feel that the only arguments that can fairly be advanced in an essay are those that are supported within the literature. This appears to suggest that the only valid form of knowledge is that which has been published. In truth, a significant amount of evidence remains unpublished and this includes some research findings, audits of practice and observations made in practice. There are different sorts of evidence and they make different contributions to a case (Pearson et al., 2007; see also Chapter 8). Before you can couple evidence with your chosen arguments, you need to ascertain how powerful the evidence is and whether it clearly supports the point that you wish to make. A poorly selected piece of evidence can undermine your essay.

Activity 9.4   *Critical thinking*

Look at the following examples of evidence coupled with arguments that you might include within an essay on interpreting healthcare policy. Determine whether you think the evidence supports the chosen argument. Then decide which one of the following examples of evidence–argument pairings seems too unconvincing to include in an essay (we share our ideas on that question at the chapter end). Finally, turn to our webpage to examine some examples of argument and evidence coupling that operate at different levels of critical thinking (**www.sagepub.co.uk/price_harrington**). When you also look at Stewart's example analytical essay on the webpage, can you see him coupling arguments and evidence there?

1. **The argument**: Nurses are confident enough to examine policies critically, blending these with care philosophy to produce care that is workable and remains within the spirit of best practice.
   The evidence: A conference paper presented by two nurse philosophers arguing that nurses have improved as discerning and articulate practitioners and are able to determine what is beneficial, realisable and effective. The nurse philosophers report their grounded theory research, which included interviews with, and observations of, nurses in practice.

continued ...

2. **The argument**: Nurses have been successful in advancing some areas of the chosen policy and delaying others, reflecting local circumstances and needs.

   The evidence: The International Council of Nurses has presented a series of findings on the role of the nurse as change agent.

3. **The argument**: There are standard care pathways that constrain healthcare professions, limiting the choices that practitioners can make.

   The evidence: Two standard care pathways in operation in local clinical areas are cited as examples of situations where practitioners sometimes express their frustration.

Our reflections are given at the end of the chapter.

Deciding which arguments and evidence make it into your essay is critical. You may have previously encountered essay feedback where the tutor has told you that your account was 'too superficial'. You are likely to be guilty of this if you try to include too many arguments and pieces of evidence. Evidence needs to be introduced and *you* need to make points about it. The exasperated assessor might observe, 'You seem to record everyone else's opinion, but not to synthesise these or to arrive at a perspective of your own!' This is often a problem where you are not thinking critically enough, showing due regard to the specific circumstances alluded to within the essay question or else you have not applied your points to a care location. Remember, higher-order critical reasoning shows greater precision; it is contextualised as well as inquisitive. Fewer carefully chosen arguments, and being more selective about what evidence you use to support them, will often stand your work in good stead.

Speculating successfully

Something that students find very difficult to achieve within an essay is speculation. If arguments are founded upon evidence, and evidence is contradictory or even absent, how do we proceed? We are left to rehearse what could be happening or what might be done next. We need to identify what can be suggested, whether that is within the literature or as part of clinical experience. We also need to imagine the future, how services might change, what patient needs could be, and how we might work better with relatives. Speculation is an important part of higher level critical thinking. Nursing practice needs nurses who are confident and willing to speculate, to imagine what might be the case, what could be required. Failing to ask the right questions often means that opportunities for improvements in practice are lost. In Table 3.1 (pages 48–9), independent thinking (the highest level of critical thought), imaginative new questions are asked of care situations. Refresh your understanding of this by turning back to Table 3.1 if you need to.

To speculate with confidence we need to use terms that signal to the reader that we have moved into speculative mode. We no longer argue something, or describe it, and we no longer claim it as fact – we speculate about it. If we signal these matters clearly and then write in a measured way about the subject (i.e., without stating what we think is 'obvious' or 'self-evident', or what 'naturally follows'), we will be taking the reader along with us, reasoning at our side.

The following words or short phrases all signal that we are speculating.

- **Notionally**: This suggests that we are considering an embryonic idea – one still in development. At this stage, the idea is still a possibility; for example: 'Notionally, nurses do more to interpret policies than they realise. Even simple care involves interpreting what equals quality.'

- **Arguably**: This is used to suggest that the point is sufficiently clear and coherent to constitute an argument, but it is one we are still considering; for example: 'Nurses' frustration with policy is arguably to do with constraints on professional freedom. Nurses object to too many limits being set on their clinical decision making.'

- **We might speculate**: This is a tentative way of putting things, suggesting an area of enquiry or a line of reasoning; for example: 'We might speculate that, while standard care plans save nurses' time, they also limit thinking. Where might I write about these concerns? There doesn't seem to be a box for that!'

- **A number of possibilities present**: This sets out possible explanations; for example: 'A number of possibilities present: first, that colleagues insist on writing their own policies; second, that they form alliances with the policy makers; and, third, that they lament change and continue to complain.'

- **It would be possible to suggest**: This hints that what is written about next has some credibility; for example: 'It would be possible to suggest that nurses are shaping the policies that matter – those that determine the experience of care.'

- **Conceivably**: This suggests something that could be considered, but might not be the easiest explanation; for example: 'Conceivably, nurse entrepreneurs are those who see policy as a lever. They use it to achieve desirable ends.'

Activity 9.5   *Reflection*

Look back over some past essays and note whether you used any of the above words or phrases to indicate that you were speculating. Did you use the words in the right way? What happens if you use them too frequently in an essay? On our web page (**www.sagepub.co.uk/price_harrington**), we offer some examples of successful speculative paragraphs, as well as some that falter, and we explain the differences between the two.

Reaching successful conclusions

A large majority of analytical essays written by students describe what has gone before within the essay, but without necessarily demonstrating a conclusion. To use a simple analogy, we describe a journey made (we spent three hours on the train). What is usually required within an analytical essay is to determine the significance of that journey. We can illustrate this by referring to the three purposes of analytical essays described earlier.

- The journey was arduous, took longer than expected and prompted us to reconsider the advantages of using public transport in the future (evaluative).

- There remain opportunities to improve upon the journey, at least with regard to the time taken. Weekday public transport schedules are better (strategic).

- Travelling by public transport had the advantage of reducing our carbon footprint. Had we driven there, the environmental penalty would have been higher (philosophical).

A successful conclusion, then, must capture the account of what has been written so far (the journey), but must also include a deduction. We have to make clear what matters seem settled and what remain open at the end of the essay. Contrary to what some students think, it is not always true that we have to have 'nailed our colours to the mast', either wholeheartedly adopting or rejecting the case presented to us in a question. We do, however, have to have clarified our position. The case seems supportable to this extent, but what we need to ascertain further is x y z.

In the following example of a concluding paragraph relating to the essay on policy interpretation, there is a clear indication of the author's resting position at the end. Notice how the author refers back to the case that has already been introduced at the start of the essay:

At the start of this paper, I introduced the case that nurses do interpret policies, but cautioned that their success in this is affected by factors that limit their freedom to proceed at will. The paper has noted that pressure of time and the need to serve a public, as well as individual patients, to work effectively in teams and to attend to employer agendas, all help determine the extent to which the nurse interprets policy. My chosen policy (rehabilitation) espouses a philosophy of cooperation and consultation. It remains an optimistic policy, at least where relatives' expectations are high and where the nurse must compromise, sharing care between patients. Nurses might wish to interpret this policy as an opportunity to deliver individualised care, but they do not always have the scope to proceed in that way. Instead, the need to ration their expertise and attention serves to contain just how much consultation they engage in.

In this conclusion, the journey is summed up quickly in the sentence describing what limits nurses' opportunities to interpret policy. The telling point arrives at the end, where it is explained that the nurse might wish to interpret policy in a particular way (as individualised care), but that care is necessarily rationed. The nurse does a little for the many and not as much as might be wished for the few. The author defends the opening case.

Activity 9.6 — Group work

It is possible to practise the formulation of conclusions as part of a conversation with your colleagues. Working with three others, have the first colleague select a subject for the imaginary essay. The second should then briefly describe the case to be made there, and the third should summarise what the conclusion is (the case might or might not be supported). The fourth colleague should then determine whether the conclusion sounded convincing. Take it in turns to play different roles, choosing another essay subject, case and conclusion, and allowing all to practise their judgements.

Drafting the essay and checking its clarity

Students vary in their preferred ways of writing and editing. Having prepared an outline plan that signals the key sections of the paper, the arguments and evidence that will appear in each, the case that will be considered and the position adopted, some quickly set down a first draft. Students may have checked that they remain within the word counts they have allocated for each section, but they will leave the references, tables or quotations to be added later. The first goal for such students is to get work down on paper that captures their understanding of the subject and that represents their position regarding it. Other students move much more incrementally, carefully crafting each section and adding embellishments as they go. However you proceed, though, checking the clarity and coherence of what has been written remains a responsibility.

We asked our four students about their essay drafting and reviewing processes.

Gina: *If you write a 'rough' draft of your essay in one sitting, you have the advantage that you don't pause to fret over doubts as you go. These will return to you later, though. Have I made this point clear, can I argue that, given what this article says?*

Fatima: *I work with my plan, especially as regards the word allowance. If one section seems tight, and I need to include more words than I thought at first, I stop right then and ask whether I'm trying to include too much. It makes editing much easier.*

Raymet: *I write first draft essays in the morning and then talk the content of my essay through with a friend. I explain what I am arguing. If they seem clear about my thoughts, even if they don't agree with my position, I feel encouraged.*

Stewart: *Writing for me is private, but I always leave several days to complete an edit. My later essays have been better for that. I say to myself, 'This isn't my essay, it's someone else's. I am going to pick it to pieces to see if it stands up.'*

We agree with Gina that doubts can creep in as you write. It is so easy to see multiple perspectives on a subject. Sometimes work grinds to a halt if you do not write a little more quickly and freely in the first instance. There is something to be said, then, for writing a first complete but more rudimentary draft. It probably captures your position most cleanly, provided that you have allocated enough thinking time before starting work.

Fatima's approach is much more 'sculpted'. The work proceeds in sections and each is 'got right' before the next is attempted. The approach does produce work that has well-balanced sections, each with a complement of words, arguments and evidence. It works well if you like to think in a stepwise fashion: 'This is what I must explain first; these are the context points. Next, I must set out the case and suggest how my essay will examine that.' Students sometimes discover their position shifting a little as they write in this way. It is then necessary to check what is claimed in the introduction – do you still support that?

We especially support Raymet's strategy of summarising a first draft essay. Notice that Raymet sticks to her guns once she has identified what her position will be. This is commendable, *provided* you have heard and considered the questions and challenges posed by others. Your friend might not have read what you have or attended the lectures that you did, so their position on a subject cannot be yours. Against that, naive questions and thoughtful challenges from reviewers are valuable, as you might well have missed something. To avoid charges of academic collusion and dishonesty, resist the temptation to ask them to edit your essay. This should remain your own work.

Stewart makes a good point when he describes how he distances himself from his own work at review stage. This is a fine example of evaluative critical thinking put to good use. The more you can imagine yourself as an editor, and less as the anxious author, the more likely you are to make the adjustments that help your work appear polished.

If you have left insufficient time to review work, or are preparing several papers in quick succession, essay editing can seem a bit of a chore. It is tempting to submit the work and hope. Time spent checking, however, is beneficial in several ways. You can:

- conduct the spelling, syntax and other presentational checks;
- ensure that the work answers the question or attends to the task set;
- assure yourself that a case has been made – one that is supported, rejected or seen as conditional within the conclusion;
- recount the arguments made and the evidence used ('Do they work together?').

Chapter summary

Each individual essay is a work that operates in context, attending to the question or task set. Even though this is an academic work, it still expresses your preferred ways of working. You are the person who drafts the work and you write in a way that enables you to present scripts on time. There are, however, certain features of good analytical essay writing that show your critical thinking at work. You need to be very clear about the purpose of the essay and to write in the appropriate way. Are you going to evaluate or philosophise, for example? You need to determine what case is being discussed and what position you take on it. In some instances, an examiner will set the case by making an assertion that you are invited to evaluate. In other instances, you select a case of your own – one that you will defend using arguments and evidence as your essay unfolds. Good analytical essay writing includes sufficient arguments and pieces of evidence to make a clear case. There is a balance struck between analytical writing (what I think) and descriptive writing (what I report). Where the debate remains open and the best way forward is still to be discovered, you will make selective use of more speculative forms of writing. Conclusions are arranged in such a way that they do more than describe what has been discussed in the text. They indicate where your reasoning has led. All of this is improved where you allocate sufficient time to editing your own work.

Activities: Brief outline answers

Activity 9.1: Critical thinking (page 144)

1. This is a tricky one. There are ethical/philosophical issues at stake here, surrounding human and reproductive rights, so the essay has a philosophical purpose. It is strategic too, though, as challenges in this instance seem to pose the question, 'What will you do next?' In these instances, the clues to what may be required often exist in the case study.
2. The purpose here is evaluative and the opening assertion, about nurses interpreting policy, makes this clear. Do you support this case?
3. The purpose here is strategic. The essay requires you to write about how you might involve lay consultants in the business of care delivery.

Activity 9.3: Critical thinking (page 145)

One plan that we have found workable is as follows.

- Essay purpose: what is asked of me?
- Case made: mine or the examiner's (name it)?
- My position: for or against the case, caveats noted.
- Section 1: introduction and signposting.
- Section 2: main body.
- Key arguments and paired evidence (argument 1, evidence; argument 2, evidence; etc.).
- Section 3: conclusions.

Activity 9.4: Critical thinking (pages 146–7)

1. The evidence here consists of research findings, but findings that might not have been published within the press. Research evidence is often thought of as more important than other forms; in this case, we would have felt more confident about it if the conference paper had to pass a peer review process before it was accepted. There seems to be a close connection made here to the argument that has to be supported.
2. Here, the evidence consists of something published by an august international body and one that, on this occasion, discusses change agency. Quite abstract points are made about nurses' change agency work and it is not certain that there is a clear connection to the policy interpretation under question (there are many forms of change). This, then, would be the argument–evidence pairing that we might sacrifice in a shortened essay.
3. The evidence here is experiential and refers to local standard care pathways. It is clearly authentic to practice, as it deals with the same environments where the policy is being interpreted. There seems to be a potentially good fit between evidence and argument.

Further reading

Gimenez, J (2011) *Writing for Nursing and Midwifery Students*, 2nd ed. Basingstoke: Palgrave Macmillan.

This accessible textbook is suitable for nurses on pre- and post-registration courses. It illustrates a wide range of writing forms, although connections to forms of thinking are not so well developed.

Greetham, B (2013) *How to Write Better Essays*, 3rd ed. Basingstoke: Palgrave Macmillan.

While this accessible text is not written specifically for nurses, it takes you through the essay planning process. There is a strong emphasis on personal organisation and preparation, as is common within such textbooks.

Hutchfield, K (2010) *Information Skills for Nursing Students*. Exeter: Learning Matters.

Several chapters from this textbook offer useful additional information. Chapter 5 offers guidance on writing skills (being literate) and Chapter 6 on technology skills (much of your writing will be sourced and prepared here). Those writing papers involving statistics or calculations might also draw upon Chapter 3, which concerns number skills for nursing practice.

Taylor, D (2014) *Writing Skills in Nursing and Healthcare: A guide to completing successful dissertations and theses.* London: Sage.

Theses and dissertations are usually associated with postgraduate courses of study. Nonetheless, wherever there is a substantial project to be submitted, this book has something to offer. The work covers everything from researching the literature, through setting out the dissertation or thesis to promulgating results at conference or seminar.

Useful websites

http://en.wikibooks.org/wiki/Writing_Better_University_Essays

Writing Better University Essays

This free to access electronic book provides a good array of guidance on essay writing in coursework and examination contexts. Although not specifically aimed at healthcare students, the guidance usually holds good as regards principles of analytical writing. The work was updated in 2014.

www.latrobe.edu.au/students/learning/develop-skills/writing

Very few 'how to' guides get much beyond the technical aspects of writing the critical essay, but Kate Chanock takes you through the ideas-formulation stages and the mustering of the same into a paper. The illustrated work isn't from nursing, it's part of the history of Australia, but the principles of good reasoning are made well enough to make this useful for nursing scholars too.

While university rules usually dictate that students taking nursing courses are articulate in written English, we believe that there is value in returning to some simple videos that refresh you on the most basic tenets of writing. YouTube has a number of these, which are easily found by typing a search: *essay writing YouTube*. Two examples are:

www.youtube.com/watch?v=2_pZWdF7ujA

How to Write a Basic Paragraph

This very simple presentation takes you through the basics of what a paragraph consists of. Much of what demonstrates critical thinking in action is provided at the level of paragraphs. You must understand the basic structure of a paragraph if you are to develop arguments clearly. This demonstration is extremely basic but, if you have been criticised for poor paragraph structure, then it may still be of benefit.

www.youtube.com/watch?v=liyFKUFCQno

How to Write a Good Essay

This demonstration focuses on how to write a good essay and it is a refreshing and, at times, amusing way to recall the tenets of essay writing. The presenter puts his information across with enthusiasm. Interestingly, he refers to a 'crunch' paragraph towards the end of the essay, just before the conclusion. This often works well, but we would encourage you to see essays not necessarily in such 'win or lose' the debate terms. In health care, the case is often a calmer appraisal of what we do and do not yet know.

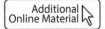 Additional Online Material

For examples of analytical essays and other useful material, please visit the companion website at **www.sagepub.co.uk/price_harrington**

Chapter 10
Writing the reflective essay

NMC Standards for Pre-registration Nursing Education

This chapter addresses the following competencies.

Domain 1: Professional values

8. All nurses must practise independently, recognising the limits of their competence and knowledge. They must reflect on these limits and seek advice from, or refer to, other professionals where necessary.

Domain 4: Leadership, management and team working

4. All nurses must be self-aware and recognise how their own values, principles and assumptions may affect their practice. They must maintain their own personal and professional development, learning from experience, through supervision, feedback, reflection and evaluation.

Chapter aims

After reading this chapter, you will be able to:

*   identify the important tasks to be attended to when writing a reflective essay;
*   discuss the functions of the reflective essay and how this affects its construction;
*   explain clearly the purpose of reflective essays;
*   demonstrate insights into the reporting of events, feelings, perceptions, perspectives, interpretations, conclusions and planned next actions associated with reflection;
*   use a chosen reflective framework in ways that help you to demonstrate your learning more clearly;
*   constructively criticise essay construction, using the case-study example provided on the companion website for this book (**www.sagepub.co.uk/price_harrington**).

Introduction

It is in the nature of nursing that we need to reflect and to be able to write reflectively. Nurses deal with human experience: concerning health and illness, linked to diagnosis and prognosis, and attendant on difficult healthcare decisions. There are sometimes no trite 'right solutions' in health care, only best reasoned and argued courses of action, founded to a significant extent upon reflection (Wyer et al., 2014). It is because nurses need to access their experience in a clear and consistent way, and because we need to understand the process of reviewing and evaluating experience, that reflection and reflective writing are so important.

Reflection is also important if we are to manage successfully the stresses of nursing care (Dolan et al., 2012). We must judge, for instance, the right level of closeness to maintain with patients, many of whom are distressingly sick. Our work is demanding, especially where we have discovered that we believe different things from other people, who may define care differently, value different goals and count other things as dignified and desirable. Our nursing work sometimes exposes us to conflict, disagreement and debate, so it is vital that we are able to make sense of such events if we are to continue caring in an open, sensitive way. We need to be aware of what we believe and value; we need to respect the beliefs of others if we are to practise well (Mason et al., 2014). Reflection is important to our wellbeing and to the preservation of a professional purpose in what we do. Table 3.2 (pages 50–1) details the different expressions of reflective reasoning as you move from absolutist thinking through transitional and contextual thinking and on to the deepest introspection within independent thinking.

In this chapter, we examine a series of key tasks associated with the business of writing reflectively, tasks linked to reflective writing coursework. Understanding these tasks will help you to write in ways that seem clearer and more coherent to others. Next, we give consideration to the reflective frameworks that you might be invited to use within your coursework. These vary by college and course, but there are certain common principles. All these frameworks ask you to attend to feelings, meanings and then actions. Finally, we turn to different levels of critical reflection, first introduced in Table 3.2 (pages 50–1). This is a relatively new area as, until recently, it was considered that either you were or you were not reflective. Levels of reflection were less discussed; at best, they were simply described in terms of students' ability to summarise events and render an account of their deductions (Padden, 2013, discusses an assessment scale of this type). In practice (and importantly for assessment), we argue that there are gradations of reflection with levels reaching well beyond description and summary of events. We discuss these levels of reflective reasoning last, referring you to Raymet's example reflective essay and example paragraphs of reflective reasoning at different levels within the companion website for this book (**www.sagepub. co.uk/price_harrington**).

Five key tasks of reflective writing

Irrespective of whether your reflective writing takes the form of a coursework essay, a report from a clinical practice placement, a case study of care planned and delivered, or a review of clinical decisions made, there are a number of tasks your work should attend to.

Representing enquiry

Reflection is a form of enquiry that sees you return to experience, delve into attitudes and values or explore the possibilities of practice. As we have seen in Chapter 2, reflection may happen while you are in action (delivering care) or after action (when you take a retrospective view). In the first of these instances, your reflections are more likely to be formative, less well developed and without the benefit of hindsight. You will need to show the reader how you are speculating about what is happening, something we touched on in Chapter 9. All reflective writing, however, needs to explain quickly the purpose and the process of the enquiry in which you are engaged. Setting up these explanations at the start of your written work will help readers to review your work with greater insight and be more appreciative of what you achieve there. As we will see below, you can only demonstrate higher level reflective reasoning, contextual thinking, if there is a clear purpose or context to your writing.

Activity 10.1   *Communication*

We asked Fatima and Gina to share with us some of the opening paragraphs they have written at the start of reflective essays. Then we asked them to summarise these into a clear purpose and process for each. Their summaries are provided below. Read each of these and then prepare brief notes on why working on such summaries might improve your reflective essay writing.

Fatima: *The purpose of this essay is to explore the ways in which I negotiated care with a family supporting a dying patient. To that end, I arrange my reflections using a series of headings, those first associated with my assumptions and perceptions of care needs, those I believed that the family held, and then the compromises that were sought as we tried to bring our expectations of care together. This is my narrative, what I thought I was engaged in when looking after others.*

Gina: *The purpose of this essay was to uncover some of the values, beliefs and aspirations that I hold with regard to holistic care. This work involved critical reflections regarding what each element of holistic care entails, and what my skills and work capacity could reasonably deliver on. My reflections conclude with a summary of the discrepancies that remain, between what I believe I should deliver and what I succeed in assisting patients with.*

Distinguishing between facts, perspectives, perceptions, narratives and discourses

Reflective writing deals with facts (e.g., the dosage of a drug taken) but it also deals regularly with perspectives and perceptions. We need to show that we appreciate distinctions between these within our work. A perspective is something that sums up our position, values, aspirations and beliefs. It is closely associated with attitude, our disposition to think of things in an enduring way (Maio and Haddock, 2009). For example, 'Care should be patient centred, working with the individual's needs' is an expression of a perspective. It is often used to describe what we think should be the case or what should happen. A perception, though, is much more fragile than this and describes the impressions that we take from incomplete or fragmentary experience. 'Mrs Jones was confused by the news; she seemed to search for words to express all the worries that suddenly arose inside her' is an example of a perception. We have no direct proof of what Mrs Jones felt, as she has not told us, but we infer that her behaviour and hesitant words were indicative of anxiety.

In some instances, you may have access to a patient or colleague narrative under development, the story that they use to explain what is happening and what they are trying to do. Narratives are a way of organising perceptions so that they make personal sense (Brown et al., 2012). Where narratives are combined and perhaps shared with others to explain more complex interactions (e.g., the process of rehabilitating after an injury), we refer to *discourses*. Discourses capture the nature and the purpose of activity, the bigger issues that are involved in health care (e.g., leadership, power, empowerment, therapy). Discourses frequently evaluate activity undertaken, so a discourse might be about improvement or failure, success or confusion. They may be overtly political, relating to what parties involved believe should happen. You may already be familiar with discourses in healthcare that help to explain why something has not worked as well as you hoped. A lack of resources is a frequently used discourse.

Much of what we reflect upon in essays revolves around facts, perceptions and perspectives. A number of mistakes are easily possible as we draft our work.

- We may allow our perspective to dominate how we imagine others think or feel (they must be like me, believe what I believe, value what I value).

- We may infer perspectives held by others based on quite limited perceptions of what they do or say (we, as it were, fill in the gaps, explaining to ourselves why others act as they do).

- We may build a perspective on a subject based on a series of perceptions, each of which is reasonable in and of itself, but which collectively become more suspect as we string these together. We over-extend our critical reflection, claiming more than seems reasonable. There is a risk that the narratives and the discourses we identify come more from our beliefs and values than a careful scrutiny of the accounts shared by others, or an examination of the behaviour witnessed.

- We muddle perception and fact, writing about perceptions *as* fact. In this instance, we forget how transient or tentative our impressions are, and we allow ourselves to feel more sure about something than is justified.

When you review the bullet points above, you should realise that many of these mistakes are associated with lower levels of reflective reasoning (Table 3.2, pages 50–1). Allowing your perspective to dominate how you imagine others think or feel is an absolutist way of thinking. You have not yet paused to imagine that there could be other perspectives, a different combination of experiences to be taken into account. Deducing something from insufficient information or a failure to consider how all the factors affecting a situation might affect experiences and outcomes, suggests quite rudimentary transitional thinking. Yes, you are aware of relevant factors, but you have filled in the gaps prematurely to reach a conclusion, perhaps one that feels more familiar or comfortable? Reflection usually requires us to explore some more, to imagine issues and concerns, to conduct what we described as speculation within Chapter 9.

To write successfully it is necessary to be clear about whether you are writing about a fact, a perspective, a perception, a narrative or a discourse. In many of the best reflective essays, nurses write about competing narratives or discourses, ways in which individuals and groups understand events. They recount their first impressions of a situation, describe how this changes, and speculate about the perceptions that others may have regarding the situation. Rather than close that debate, arguing that this or that is therefore the case, they acknowledge that the situation remains ambiguous and that further interpretation is needed. Here is a successful example of that from Gina's work on holistic care:

Spiritual care was challenging for me, as I typically associated it with religious belief and especially my religious beliefs. So my default perspective was that, to talk about spiritual care was to talk about how others live their religious convictions. It seemed apparent, though, that other people, including those who were not overtly religious, also had a sense of the spiritual. This appeared to be associated with that which was aesthetic, beautiful, meaningful, especially as regards good living in its different guises. I discovered that it was about that which made people feel dignified and good about themselves, about that which made them more than a role, someone with a purpose as well as a function in society. It was about what they described as 'me'. Some patients had a different narrative regarding what it means to be spiritual and it was just as powerful for them as my religious convictions were for me.

The key point here, then, is do not confuse the reader regarding what you are writing about. Distinguish clearly between terms such as perception and perspective, and use these terms consistently. A glossary of key terms used may also help the reader.

Demonstrating insight

In many instances, reflective writing requires you to take a risk to share with the reader some insights into your beliefs, ways of thinking and operating. At best, these insights demonstrate your quizzical attitude towards what you do or believe. In Table 3.2 (pages 50–1), independent thinking (the highest standard of reflection) relating to the understanding of yourself, involves seeing 'experience as an opportunity to re-examine the nurse's [your] own values, beliefs and attitudes. The account shows the nurse questioning that in her or himself that affects their expertise, their readiness or their fit to particular elements of practice.' It can feel uncomfortable to write in this way, especially if you fear that the examiner will condemn you for what you have not achieved. In a healthcare culture that expects consistency and excellence, perhaps beyond human or system capacity, it is more difficult to confide things about what seemed imperfect within yourself and have remained open to improvement or revision. We explain what is involved in becoming more critical in your reflections below, but this always involves some increasing introspection.

To help you to share insights more openly, it is worth checking with your tutor in advance that the essay is being assessed as evidence of continued learning and professional growth. Well-written assign-ment briefs should make this apparent from the outset, although you should note caveats about professional standards. To confide that you have behaved in an unprofessional or illegal manner may still mean that the work triggers some form of sanction. The reflective essay is not a confessional that absolves you of all guilt for acts that have been dangerous or demeaning for patients.

The important point here is first to liaise with your tutor to check the purpose of the reflective essay set. Then, when it is clear that you should evaluate your own practice and reasoning, pick out what you have assumed, what requires further attention. The writing does not need to seem revelatory, to the extent that you will now completely transform all that you do. Such a transfor-mation probably requires many introspective investigations into your habitual ways of thinking and working. But it should demonstrate insight, a clearer understanding of what now seems problematic, incomplete, less considered or sensitive, or perhaps what has been successful and especially effective. Remark upon the next work you will do, which you will attend to more or differently in order to conduct patient-centred care.

Activity 10.2   *Reflection*

Pause to write a short passage of reflective work in which you express doubts about your own reasoning or decision making. Alternatively, use the passage to explore what might be incomplete or incoherent in your care philosophy, much as Gina does in Activity 10.1 above. Try to determine where you have thought too narrowly, a little naively or without reference to some important information.

When you have prepared this passage, turn to the example that we share at the end of this chapter and review our brief notes on what seems successful in such writing. Other passages of insight demonstration are to be found on the web page associated with this book. There, we link those passages to the different standards of reflective writing in evidence (**www. sagepub.co.uk/price_harrington**).

Respecting others

When writing reflectively, we run the risk that we express prejudices, opinions and attitudes that demonstrate a disregard for the rights and dignity of others. This is not simply a matter of political correctness; the NMC *Code* (Nursing and Midwifery Council, 2015) makes it very clear that we must have regard for the feelings and concerns of others and protect their human rights. We should not foist our perspectives on others. While you are advised in reflective essays or case studies to create pseudonyms for others discussed within your answer (protecting their identity), expressing prejudicial and unsubstantiated views about them is still likely to prompt criticism of your work. Nurses respect and support the dignity of others (Price, 2009). It is necessary to write circumspectly and to consider carefully whether expressed attitudes might signal a disregard for patients or colleagues, cause offence to the reader, or suggest that we might practise in ways that could be detrimental to nursing. This requirement relates not only to those of a different gender, age, colour, culture, religious background or sexual identity from your own, but to any with whom you have professional working relationships. Check, therefore, that what you include in your reflection demonstrates a respect for others. By all means acknowledge difference – the diversity of human experience and need – but do not assume that your own perspectives on matters are inherently superior.

Illustrating learning

Your reflective essay has one further function, and that is to demonstrate your learning. If you write in a static way, about an unquestioned perspective or perceptions that seem set in stone, you are unlikely to have attended to the last of the five tasks – the illustration of learning. Good reflective writing takes the reader on a journey, from that which is shared at the start of the essay to that which is shared at the end. In this regard, reflective writing stands in sharp contrast to other forms of academic writing. In the analytical essay, the student often creates a case and then defends that using a series of arguments within the main text (see Chapters 3 and 9). In reflective writing, however, the approach is iterative and insightful. As the paragraphs and sections unfold, the reader gains a sense of your reasoning as it changes and grows. Figure 10.1 illustrates what we mean by this, using a flow chart and some of Gina's work on holistic practice.

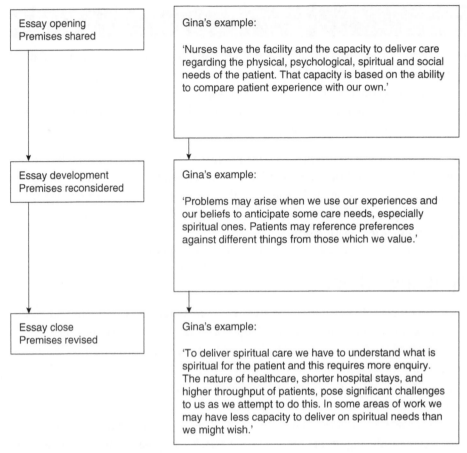

Figure 10.1: Reflecting and learning

Activity 10.3   *Critical thinking*

At the next opportunity, take a moment to revisit a piece of your own reflective writing and try to describe the movement in your thinking that you share there.

- Is there a deepening of your appreciation of the complexity of health care?
- Do you understand something new about the diversity of need?
- Do you demonstrate a process of debate under way as you consider what you encounter?

In some past essays, there may be little or no movement in your thinking and you could usefully consider what would show your learning as you wrote. In others, the movement may be inconsistent. In one passage you move towards one perspective and in another passage towards a different one. The reader cannot easily determine what you are concluding about your experiences.

- Does this suggest something important to you as regards reflecting before you write?

We share brief remarks on this last point at the end of the chapter.

Using reflective frameworks

Many students learn the process of reflective writing using one or other of the reflective practice frameworks. Ashby (2006) notes that a key benefit of using reflective frameworks or models is that we learn the discipline of seeing experiences from different perspectives. We 'frame' experiences in different ways and are then able (with colleagues) to discuss the perspectives that we develop, adopt or abandon along the way. Among the reflective frameworks commonly used within nursing courses are those proposed by Gibbs (1988) and Johns (1995). The Gibbs framework encourages us to:

1. **Clearly describe the situation**. Without premature judgement, state what happened or what we understand to be factual.
2. **Explore our feelings**. Feelings are often a filter through which we read events. Does this experience represent a threat, an accolade, a challenge or affirmation of what we do? Do feelings help me understand what was challenging, difficult, delightful or encouraging here?
3. **Evaluate the experience**. Was this positive, negative, confusing or ambiguous?
4. **Reflect**. Make sense of the experience. Do we have a chance to learn here and to confirm what counts as excellent? Is this something that helps me to understand a wider range of healthcare needs, or the consequences of action or inaction?
5. **Conclude**. What do we take away from this? Can these lessons be applied elsewhere?
6. **Act**. What we might do differently in the future?

The popular framework by Rolfe and Jasper (2010) asks the nurse to address questions in three distinct areas: *what?* (events and experiences), *so what?* (significance and consequences) and *what next?* (necessary actions or responses).

- **What?** For example, what was happening? What were my feelings and those that I surmise others had?

- **So what?** For example, what is the significance of these events? What have been or could be the consequences of this for instance.

- **What next?** For example, what remains to be done, what is now mandated? Is something urgent, do we need to change course in some way?

At their best, reflective frameworks help us to showcase our learning. As we consider matters such as the aesthetics of care, review the ways in which beliefs and feelings shaped what we did, we demonstrate both insight and change. At the end of the essay, we can state what we might do differently in the future, because we can articulate what experience has taught us in the past. Writing using the reflective frameworks, however, requires a little thought. We commend the following.

- Start by making a series of points that you wish to write about and decide under which framework heading these will appear (otherwise you might make the same point in more than one place).

- If you find that there are no points for some framework headings, decide whether this matters.

- Decide whether you wish to write about something rather bigger than the incident or care episode, perhaps relating to narratives and discourses you see developing over time with this patient. Consult your tutor on how best to do this and whether there is scope within the current essay to embark on that.

- Do not be afraid to discuss key concepts with your tutor. In reflective writing, clarity in the use of concepts and their consistent use in the essay are important. For example, are you confident in your understanding of what counts as aesthetic?

Activity 10.4   *Critical thinking*

Look at the following short care situations and decide what you think might be important using the 'what?', 'so what?' and 'what next?' questions proposed by Rolfe and Jasper (2010). Add a note explaining why each is important.

1. An angry patient visits you in the group practice and insists that it is high time that he was seen by a general practitioner rather than you in the diabetes care clinic that you run.
2. A patient confides in you that he has been having suicidal thoughts.
3. The daughter of a woman who is suffering from dementia expresses the view that it has now become critical for her mother to move into a nursing home.

Compare your answer with ours at the end of the chapter.

Levels of reflective reasoning

During the 1980s, Honey and Mumford (1982) developed their typology of learning styles, arguing that different students had different aptitudes for particular sorts of learning. No single person was a pure-type learner, they argued, but we all have propensities to learn in particular ways. To learn in another style required additional commitment and work. The four learning styles described by Honey and Mumford were *activists* (students who liked to learn through projects, practical enquiries or research), *theorists* (those who liked to build and relate new experience to existing theories), *reflectors* (those who liked to examine situations from the point of view of experience and different perspectives used there) and *pragmatists* (those who like to solve problems, to produce outcomes that were tangible and confidence boosting). Understanding learning styles is important, because it may help to explain why writing at more sophisticated reflective reasoning levels can prove so difficult. You might be excellent at writing analytical essays (theorists often excel there) but find it much harder to develop a reflective approach to experience. Those whose learning disposition is to other styles of learning have to adapt when required to write a reflective practice essay.

It can seem hard for students with other learning styles to 'reflect for reflection's sake' but, in our experience, it is possible to make headway when you give further and more familiar purpose to reflection. So the theorist might use a series of reflections to build a theory that explains particular sorts of behaviour (e.g. aggression). The activist might develop reflections that are then tested out in practice enquiry (e.g. different ways to provide reassurance). The pragmatist might be encouraged to see reflection as one of the tools in the armoury of clarifying what constitutes a healthcare problem. Importantly, that work starts at the outset with the question, does a problem exist in the first place? We would encourage assessors then to locate reflective practice essays within larger enquiries, those that have extrinsic purpose for the learner, as well as developing the powers of insight and empathy that we have alluded to above. Working with learning styles enables the students to develop their reflective practice abilities in a more confident manner.

You will need to distinguish between levels of reflection to decide whether the essay you are preparing is operating at the required level. We discuss each of the levels in turn and encourage you to examine this further by visiting the resources to be found at **www.sagepub.co.uk/price_harrington**.

Absolutist reflection (lowest level reflection)

In absolutist reasoning there is little or no introspection, little or no attention given to different interpretations of events, practice progress or goals. Instead, there is one absolute and personally reassuring perspective on care, your and others' part in that. Sometimes this is described as 'common sense'. Other competing perspectives, other options and possibilities are dismissed as misguided at best, whimsical or even destructive. Descriptions of events are described with great conviction. You are sure the perspective you have adopted is the right one. Alternatives are barely considered. In extremis, if you think in this way, you have not begun to reflect at all. You admit no doubt into your deliberations.

When we have encountered this way of thinking in students, we have explored with them some of the possible beliefs and values that underpin this viewpoint. Why does it seem hard to consider alternative perspectives, to admit to doubt within nursing practice? Here are some of the responses that we have received:

- Reflection is whimsical; it cannot bring about change and, in the meantime, we waste time and effort.

- People will always have different opinions. We cannot change those, so it is better to work on what can be proven and required.

- Reflection is just too uncomfortable to engage in. If what I think or do is not enough, not valuable, then it would be hard to carry on.

Each of these reservations has been sincerely expressed, albeit in slightly different forms and on different occasions. Without confronting such beliefs, it is much harder for you to engage in reflection and write in the way that will earn best marks. To counter the first two beliefs, it is worth considering the power of perceptions and values. Much of health care is shaped by such perceptions and values, what we and others willingly deliberate upon. Predicting behaviour can be difficult, as other people process information in different ways and with reference to different values (Connor and Norman, 2005). If you consider, for example, why patients sometimes do not follow sound medical advice, that which is evidence based, does the answer lie with the patients' values and attitudes? If they do not want to change a lifestyle in response to medical advice, is evidence enough to change matters? Yet evidence-based practice is widely applauded. What is needed is a closer examination of how patients reason and how we reason too as we guide and advise patients. If we do not understand how they and we think, there seems little prospect of effecting change. Reflection is at least as important as evidence in improving health care. Reflection is not a whimsical activity and if we understand the way in which patients construct meanings from their experience, then we can construct different ways of explaining healthcare opportunities and improvements to inspire and encourage them.

Students are candid when they confide that to admit to doubt and so many different possibilities in nursing care is uncomfortable. They operate at Benner's (2001) lowest level of reasoning, where they want there to be certainties, where rules and regulations direct care activity. It would be nice, they might reason, if all nurse education could be reduced to the learning of procedures and techniques. Yet, in clinical practice, such reassurance is rarely available. Newly registered nurses have to theorise and extemporise as they go. Patients are individuals, they behave in different ways and expect different things. Care does not proceed according to a formula. So to admit to doubt, to concede the uncertainty that afflicts some practice, is not to confide a weakness. Rather, it is to claim a strength, as long as we enquire what possible concerns, needs and interests might exercise the patient and require our response. Patients are not our adversaries but, like chess players, they do make moves, some driven by anxiety, fear or confusion, and nurses need to anticipate these responses. Reflection builds our ability to read practice situations as they develop and this is a key skill for you as a registered nurse.

Activity 10.5 — *Reflection*

Consider whether you have had doubts about reflection in any of the above ways. With regard to the three bullet points above, what might be revealed if you write about your own values, attitudes and beliefs? There are many different nursing values and attitudes and equally compassionate ones. Confide your thoughts to a trusted tutor to better understand why reflection is a risk worth taking in your written work.

Transitional reflection (low level reflection)

Transitional reflection might be thought of as a cataloguing exercise, one in which you admit that there are many points to consider, many perspectives to understand, but that you will reveal comparatively little as regards your deductions. To refer to Rolfe and Jasper's (2010) model, you are content to ask 'what?' but are rather more circumspect about confiding your deductions in 'so what?' At this level of reflection, you are less confident to draw conclusions about what a collection of observations and experiences add up to. You may be uncertain your deductions will be respected by the examiners. You may believe that others have better reasoning than you, that this comes only with experience, as nurses accumulate a large number of care episodes to draw upon.

In transitional reflection, you acknowledge a range of possibilities. You understand that care can be read in different ways and people construct their own meaning from experience. You know, for example, that pain and pain relief are intertwined experiences. The experience of pain may be mediated by the patient's expectations of pain relief. Will pain be removed altogether or simply modulated? Meaning is constructed from experience, a process applying as much to nurses as to patients, as Raymet's essay in our web resource suggests.

What is important in moving up and out of this level of reflective reasoning is a willingness to speculate. A number of deductions may follow from a series of observations in practice. None (at this stage) is proven or tested, none is absolute or reputation defining. Instead, they are possibilities – notions about what 'this might all mean'. Sharing your speculations, the tentative deductions you reach, alerts the reader to the range of possibilities you have considered. They assure the reader that you have not prematurely concluded what is happening, but you understand the need to reach some 'try it and see' explanations that you could test in practice.

Contextual reflection (higher level reflection)

Students sometimes indicate that they think of context only in clinical or patient terms. Thinking is contextualised to clinical field or role or to patient need. Contextual reflection, however, admits a wider range of contexts. It is the recognition of this that helps a marker determine that you have reflected more successfully. Here are some possible contexts:

- Your professional concerns and doubts. Reflections that attend to these, in a more transparent and inquisitive way, attract reward from the marker. Imagine that you have explained at the start of your essay that you have been concerned to understand how you listen, how you attend to everything the patient says. You then reflect on your difficulty about asking patients to clarify their expressions of concern. You do not feel you can probe into the patient's worries. Identifying this difficulty, you are reflecting contextually, with regard to the purpose of your essay.

- The nature of a problem. As suggested above, problems are defined by people; they exist when people define behaviour or care situations as problematic. If you focus your reflections in ways that attend very closely to how the problem is being defined by you and others, you are reflecting contextually.

- A change under way. There may be a shift in care or in ideas about best practice. The working relationship between the nurse and the patient may be changing, perhaps during rehabilitation. You are thinking contextually, in a more nuanced way, if you ponder experiences with close regard to that change, what characterises it and what it might mean for your work as a nurse.

Activity 10.6 — *Reflection*

Before reading on, pause to consider whether you think you have thought about context in clear enough terms in your past writing? Had you thought of context as purely to do with the patient and their needs? Remember, reflective writing might be needed in a wide variety of contexts, for example in research evidence and its use in practice. Look back to some of your reflective practice essays. How important was it to establish a focus, a purpose or a context (it is called different things?) for the reflection in the introduction to your work?

Independent reflection (highest level reflection)

The highest level of reflective reasoning is difficult to explain but we are persuaded that it is open to analysis, unlike Benner's (2001) intuition that it can be articulated. Independent reflection is characterised by an ability to treat your own beliefs and values as one influence in care, but not one with more power than others. You concede that the world of health care is a place of competing values and attitudes and that it is necessary to interrogate your own and others' attitudes to better determine how this realm of ideas, feelings and attitudes shapes how people behave. Independent reflection is, in this sense, truly philosophical; it explores issues relating to ethics, priorities, identity and meaning as care is negotiated.

We discussed this definition with Raymet and twice she confirmed that she understood it during our discussion, only for her to return later to confess that she was less sure what it meant, what it might look like in essay writing. We illustrate it in our sample paragraphs on the website, but with regard to Raymet's concerns, at the time, we suggested that she take our explanation and reword it, bringing it back for us to hear and confirm as clear and correct or otherwise. Here is Raymet's way of putting it:

> *You are reflecting independently when you're not afraid to treat yourself as a player in the scene. It is like you are an actor and you're ready to examine the play and your part in it. So you have stepped outside your role and you have asked, how is the way that I am thinking working with how others are thinking? If I am not understanding people, then I am ready to think again about what we are doing ... everything!*

The theatrical analogy works well here. Independent reflection is brave; you are willing to scrutinise your values, beliefs and attitudes and see if they fit with those of others. You are willing to pause and ask difficult questions about whether you are being as beneficial, as therapeutic, as you first thought. On the page, such writing has a startling effect. You are seeing care afresh. You dare to ask the questions others have set aside. The reflections remain focused, they are still purposeful and contextualised, but now they are refreshing. The reader is convinced that you have the insights to change practice and, while that might require the persuasion of others, you can explain what you have deduced new in the familiar care around you.

We can now summarise levels of reflective reasoning. At one extreme, there is little or no reflection present, you admit no other possibilities, explanations or perspectives to your own. The absolutist individual may well fear reflection, as it brings into focus attitudes and values that are personally cherished and which, if critically evaluated, might mean they need to shift position on issues in health care. In transitional reasoning, other possibilities and perspectives are admitted into the debate but these are kept at arm's length. The student holds back deducing what these add up to. They are cautious about exposing their position. In contextual reflective reasoning, the nurse not only does share deductions but he or she also consistently connects this to the chosen context of the reflection. The reflection is much better focused and purposeful. In independent reflective reasoning, a refreshing – sometimes even a startling – new insight is shared on the subject area; the nurse thinks in a way that she or he sees the bigger picture of a situation and can treat their own part in it in an inquisitive, evaluative and a critical way. This is the most creative, the most searching and the highest level of reflective reasoning.

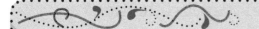

Chapter summary

Reflective writing requires just as much discipline as other forms of academic work, but it also attends to the interpretation of events and the representation of your learning, conclusions and planned next actions. You demonstrate to the reader the sense you have made of experience. Reflective writing will be clearer, more effective and more

continued ...

convincing if you are clear about the purpose of a given essay, if you use reflective frame-works consistently and transparently, and if you arrange your points under the relevant section headings of the work. Remember to be clear what you are writing about – facts, perceptions, perspectives, narratives and discourses. You may feel that you have a natural aptitude for reflection and writing about experience. Alternatively, you may feel happier writing in other ways. Reflective writing, though, is an important discipline for nurses. Much of nursing care involves deliberating on messy issues, those relating to what the patient needs or might value, or those regarding what might represent better quality care. Much as we might wish best practice to be readily defined and supported by research evidence, this is often not the case. Nurses will continue deliberating on how best to proceed and reflections upon experience remain important there. We need to represent our reflections successfully to others, to help them understand the reasoning that underpins our actions.

Activities: Brief outline answers

Activity 10.2: Reflection (page 159)

Here is my reflective paragraph, which demonstrates a measured and critical evaluation of what was discovered during a community placement. The passage relates to giving advice on nutrition to patients, some of whom do not have the financial resources to which we might be accustomed.

> *It seems possible to treat the 'well-balanced diet' as a mantra that I was all too ready to chant with patients: 'Do this, eat that and you will remain healthy.' I was repeating a formula and not stopping to examine the implications of what I said. Neville, an elderly gentleman I visited within an inner-city borough, brought me up short: 'Look lass, can you tell me what the cost is of a Sunday joint, a mix of fresh vegetables and some fruit out of season?' I shook my head; I couldn't. My comfortable lifestyle had never demanded that I pause to consider such things. 'Well,' he continued, 'I can tell you it's dearer than a packet of supermarket budget biscuits and less comforting than the bottle of stout I drink each night. Some of us exist on different things. Some of us either can't afford fresh fruit or else we prefer to sup something that gives us pleasure.' I felt mortified. I had offered Neville the textbook answer and he hadn't read my textbook. I wasn't thinking at all clearly or incisively and now I had irritated a patient who probably saw me as a middle-class busybody.*

Notice how I use quotes from the patient to capture the challenge encountered during placement. Notice, too, how I register shock at the patient's response: 'I felt mortified.' I move on to suppose how Neville might see me, reflecting on the lost opportunity to advise him on his diet in more sensitive ways. I do not condemn myself, but neither do I pull punches. I had assumed something about a patient, without sufficient information.

Activity 10.3: Critical thinking (page 160)

Our point here would be that reflective writing is both a process and a product. The very act of writing something down can trigger new insights. We learn as we write. In nursing courses, however, many such essays are products too – representations of your learning. They are assessed and graded. To that end, you should either roughly draft reflections where you can try out your insights before you prepare the essay, or else you should be prepared to go back and edit your work – not simply with regard to syntax and spelling, but with regard to arranging points that show how your thinking has changed.

Activity 10.4: Critical thinking (page 162)

1. While you are unlikely to gain anything by directly resisting a patient's requested referral to his general practitioner (GP), a key what question here is, 'what is the basis of your concern?' It may be that the patient is dissatisfied with elements of your care; he may not be familiar with all of your expertise, but

it still seems necessary to understand the felt need here. There may be a variety of reasons for such a request, including the discussion of problems that seem most comfortably discussed with a healthcare professional of the same gender for instance. So the 'what?' questions here centre on what is going on and what is the felt need. The 'so what?' questions build on what the patient feels able to disclose to you. What follows if the patient does not have confidence in my care? What follows if there are some areas of care that are best discussed with others? Have we arranged the clinic in such a way that the patient still feels adequately in contact with their GP? The 'what next?' questions might then centre on making the referral and determining what information to share with the GP. Will you express any worries that you believe the patient has with the services you provide?

2. The risks of suicide cannot be overestimated, so we would be surprised if you did anything other than raise these concerns with senior authority and record and date this information in the patient's care record. But consider the 'what' questions. Assuming that you have alerted colleagues to this expressed risk, what questions might centre on the events or circumstances that have led up to this expressed thought? Understanding the state of distress felt by a patient provides supplemental information, which might inform the monitoring of the patient and subsequent assessment of their changing state of mind. There are 'what?' questions too about the patient's appearance, demeanour, body language, all of which adds information to their expressed suicidal thoughts. What about this patient helps me to understand their state of mind now? Is the patient's expressed thought associated with anything else; for example, hallucinations? Supplemental questions might centre on the origins of these thoughts; for example, has medication been adhered to? The 'so what?' questions centre upon risk, most obviously the risk of inaction. Is a suicide attempt imminent? Can I leave this patient alone at this point? The 'what next?' questions centre around the gathering of information and conveying this accurately to those to whom you refer the patient. The questions include those about changed patterns of monitoring, the changing focus on patient mood and volition.

3. The 'what?' questions here are likely to centre on what is happening to this carer or her mother that has meant she is requesting a review of care location. 'What is going on here?' is a colloquial question, but it captures the concerns you should have. What in the patient's or daughter's circumstances have changed? Has the patient's dementia deteriorated, her behaviour changed in a way that we have not identified before? The 'so what?' questions are likely to centre on what your responsibilities are now. Do you go and investigate the situation; do you refer the patient to others; do you corroborate the daughter's report; and, if you attempt to do so, what might that mean for her assessment of you? The 'what next?' questions may well centre on further assessments of the patient and deliberations on interim support measures for the daughter. To what extent is she coping? How long can that coping continue? Has the working relationship with the daughter to now be rebuilt?

Further reading

Bolton, G (2014) *Reflective Practice: Writing and professional development*, 4th ed. London: Sage.

Reflective practice and writing is not limited to health care, so dipping into this book, which deals with the process more generally, is very valuable. Gillie Bolton's chapters on perspective and narrative are especially good.

Frank, A (2013) *The Wounded Storyteller: Body illness and ethics*, 2nd ed. Chicago, IL: University of Chicago Press.

One of the best ways into reflective practice is to glimpse what you do not understand about patients and their needs. This book helps you to do that. It introduces you to the way in which patients tell stories (narratives) to themselves to explain their own predicament to themselves.

Howatson-Jones, L (2016) *Reflective Practice in Nursing*, 3rd ed. London: Sage/Learning Matters.

This is a good source of information on reflective practice models and the process of reflecting in a methodical way. The text is accessible, practical and reassuringly 'how to'.

Useful website

On this occasion, we are directing you to one website and suggesting an exercise you might try. You can find others by conducting a search using terms such as 'patient narratives' or 'illness stories'.

www.healthstorycollaborative.org/audio-stories.html

Health Story Collaborative: Harnessing the Healing Power of Stories

This website offers you a selection of short audio recording accounts of patients' and carers' experience of illness and how they have tackled it. What is especially valuable about such narratives is that they admit you into the perceptions and the perspectives of the individuals concerned. They suggest some of the attitudes and the values they use to cope with and in many instances to overcome or transform the illness experience. To practise with greater empathy, though, we need to consider how we might use stories such as these to approach and support patients in a different way. So we recommend that with one or two colleagues you select one or more stories. After listening carefully to these, answer the following questions:

- What within this story changes my understanding of this person as a patient and the role they could play if we were planning care together?
- What within the story or stories surprised me about how patients think and what they can do?
- What within the stories mandates new questions that I should be asking patients when I first meet them and as we review their subsequent care over the days, weeks or even months ahead?
- Is there anything within the stories that shifts my sense of responsibility, of who is responsible for making something happen? If the patient shoulders a partner share in that responsibility, in what ways can this liberate how I communicate with patients?
- How can I narrate my reflections here, so the reader understands what I am enquiring about and what in consequence I speculate upon?

| Additional Online Material | For examples of analytical essays and other useful material, please visit the companion website at **www.sagepub.co.uk/price_harrington** |

Chapter 11
Building and using your portfolio of learning

NMC Standards for Pre-registration Nursing Education

This chapter addresses the following competencies.

Domain 1: Professional values

7. All nurses must be responsible and accountable for keeping their knowledge and skills up to date through continuing professional development. They must aim to improve their performance and enhance the safety and quality of care through evaluation, supervision and appraisal.

Domain 3: Nursing practice and decision making

1. All nurses must use up-to-date knowledge and evidence to assess, plan, deliver and evaluate care, communicate findings, influence change and promote health and best practice.

Chapter aims

After reading this chapter, you will be able to:

- discuss the best ways to set out a portfolio;
- appreciate the advantages of building a portfolio;
- identify the ways in which you are thinking critically as you compile and use your portfolio;
- suggest ways in which individual reflections can be built on through the portfolio;
- identify a range of circumstances under which drawing excerpts from your portfolio might enable you to make a case about either your development or your professionalism.

Introduction

Portfolios of learning, learning journals or logs and personal professional profiles are used widely within higher education and the nursing profession beyond, to help students organise a coherent account of their achievements, enquiries and development (Reed, 2015). They combine hard evidence of experience (e.g., a practice placement record) with reflexive evidence of learning (e.g., a series of structured reflections on what has been discovered).

In 2015, the Nursing and Midwifery Council made important changes to revalidation, the process by which nurses demonstrate their continuing fitness to practice (**www.nmc.org.uk/ standards/revalidation**). All nurses are now required to demonstrate in each three-year period a minimum of 40 hours of continuing professional development (of which 20 must be open to confirmation by others), they must have created five pieces of work that demonstrate consultation with service recipients (receiving feedback on their practice), and they must demonstrate a minimum of five written reflections on *The Code*, all discussed with another nurse prepared to confirm their achievements. The confirmation process is envisaged as logically running as part of the annual appraisal activity completed by nurses in their workplaces. While a portfolio is not dictated as the record system for these achievements, it is clear that nurses will need some sort of reflective record. Simple attendance at study days, for example, will not count as reflective learning. So portfolio work not only has currency in nursing courses, it is important as part of registered nurse practice beyond.

While the term used to describe such records may vary slightly from setting to setting, the rationale remains the same. The portfolio exists to represent nurses' development over time, the areas they have enquired into and what they have deduced or mastered there. The portfolio allows the nurse to make a case not only about what has been learned but also why this is relevant to their practice and, in the case of students, how course learning outcomes have been met. In the future, portfolios have the potential to help to audit trail longer enquiries, those into the narratives of patients and practitioners over time, or the discourses that shape the nature of health care. There is no reason, for instance, why the portfolio might not constitute a major record of work conducted towards a doctoral thesis.

This chapter sets out guidance on the building and the use of a portfolio as part of your professional work as a nurse. It highlights the part that critical and reflective thinking play. You are encouraged to read this in conjunction with any course or university requirements relating to the format of the portfolio. For example, in some instances this will be a hard-copy document that you carry with you to interviews and placements. In other situations, it may be an electronic document or even a collection of documents stored within your personal space on the course website. In building and presenting your portfolio, it is necessary to remain mindful of the requirements set down by the university or professional organisation that reviews such work.

Portfolio building is not something to which all nurses turn eagerly. Unlike an artist, who must show a portfolio of work to gain new commissions or exhibition opportunities month by month, registered nurses are only periodically required to illustrate their achievements. We are not all diary keepers or plan makers in the sense that portfolios facilitate. Nonetheless, the portfolio skills that you develop on your course will stand you in good stead later, not only to help you pass assessments but also to make a best case regarding your credentials when you apply for a new job or promotion, or make an application to a postgraduate course. Portfolios of learning can sometimes enable you to claim accreditation for prior experiential learning, shortening the length of study you need to do in subsequent courses, or gaining you entry into a course where you do not hold the best fit entry qualifications.

> ### Activity 11.1   *Reflection*
>
> Take a moment to reflect why portfolio evidence of learning might be advantageous in your career. Consider the emphasis placed on competency and evidence-based practice in nursing today. Consider what messages about your organisational ability and communication skills can successfully be conveyed to readers using a portfolio. Recounting such advantages and writing them down as bullet points as a motivating aide memoire in the front of your portfolio can help you to persevere with your portfolio building in the months ahead.

Choosing or designing a portfolio of your own

While some universities issue students with a formatted learning log that they are required to use, most allow the student carte blanche to develop one of their own, provided that it complies with certain requirements. At a minimum, this means that there is space for a record of experience and courses or modules completed (here you may keep a record of clinical placements, visits, projects or field trips conducted); a place where you reflect on what your experience, teaching or enquiry has taught you (this section usually requires that you relate your insights to course learning outcomes); and a space where you can write up your aims and strategies for further enquiry (this is the prospective part of the portfolio and provides a chance for you to demonstrate your strategic thinking). In theory, then, a portfolio can be successfully built using a looseleaf folder and some dividing cards to enable you to create sections within your work. Alternatively, you might set it up as a folder within your computer with files arranged under each of the key sections. What is important is that, whatever format your portfolio takes, it should be:

- logically arranged and accessible (with sections and contents pages);
- consistently arranged (e.g., using standard sections, subsections and headings);
- well presented (avoiding spelling and syntax errors; communication is important in this area of nursing, as in all others);
- up to date and representative of your learning (records that stopped several months ago prompt questions about what you have done more recently).

For students who have access to an electronic learning space associated with their course, there are real advantages in keeping an electronic portfolio. The advantage of this format is that you can readily update or change your entries, building and representing evidence of achievement as you go along. The record is less static than if it were to be presented on a printed page but remains open to printing whenever you need it. If you use this format, however, you need to be sure that it can be downloaded to your own computer after the course is completed, as several elements of this work may be relevant to your future career. It is necessary to check the university rules on the use and privacy terms relating to this record and to respect any restrictions placed there on the nature of records that can be made.

Critical thinking and your portfolio

Portfolios consist of several different sorts of evidence arranged as a coherent whole to represent your learning. The way in which you order this evidence, relating one sort to another and linking all to your strategic plans, demonstrates a great deal about your ability to conceptualise (e.g., identifying problems and learning needs), to analyse (e.g., what seemed to be possible ways forward) and to strategise (e.g., selecting the right enquiries to make). Remember, independent thinking and the ability to contextualise your learning to a strategic plan are very much part of the higher levels of reasoning that you read about in Chapter 3 of this book. The highest levels of reflective reasoning, those which critique values and attitudes and demonstrate increasing creativity, might also be exhibited through a series of entries within your portfolio. A simple arrangement for the portfolio could be as shown in Table 11.1.

Portfolio section	Design notes
Preliminary section, including your name, contact details, contents list and list of key reference sources (websites, telephone numbers, email addresses)	This is a precious document, so including your name and contact details is important were it to be lost. 'Lost' here can include computer crashes, so be sure to back up your portfolio files on a regular basis, storing these in a place beyond the computer itself. Your contents list needs to include sections and then a list of all entries in each. Be consistent in your approach as you will probably need to cross-reference material within the portfolio, for example entry one within your first section becomes 1.1 and so on. Adding an aide memoire of the web addresses for key enquiry resources, and for those within the library and beyond, is also helpful as they are to hand whenever you update your portfolio.
Section 1: Evidence of achievements, courses or learning, projects or field trips completed	You need a section where you can include all the different sorts of evidence that testify to the experience you have gained. Label each entry so it corresponds to your contents list. Entries here may take different forms, and may include, for example, certificates of attendance or course completion, reference lists of reading programme papers reviewed, or copies of reports relating to clinical placements. Note that this evidence does not in itself always demonstrate learning. Simply listing articles read doesn't tell us what you deduce from your reading. You will therefore need to either add short reflective annotations to some entries, or cross-reference the entry in your next section where you write up your reflections more extensively. Because your portfolio needs to remain a 'live and current document', it will be periodically necessary to replace some very old pieces of evidence with that which has superseded it. Were this not to be the case, you would have a portfolio in several volumes and with some early entries of only historical interest. Check with your tutor before doing this on a course. Here evidence is not usually replaced until course end.

(Continued)

(Continued)

Portfolio section	Design notes
Section 2: Evidence of reflection and debate, and the meanings that you ascribe to experience	Each entry in this section is likely to be referenced against one or more course learning outcomes and to use the reflective framework that you have chosen or that has been required by the college. Evidence here may relate to clinical experience, reflections upon workshop activities or seminars, debates that have arisen after a lecture or observations made after shadowing a more experienced practitioner. Wherever experience offers a constructive learning opportunity there is scope to make an entry. Remember that reflections are not necessarily one to one – a reflection for each individual experience. Sometimes you will write reflections relating to a series of experiences. This is why a system of cross-referencing is important.
Section 3: Plans, future aims and learning strategies	You might expect this section to appear at the front of the portfolio but, as learning is incremental and plans are frequently revised, we suggest that it appears at the end. The wording of your entries here is important. Try to ensure that you are specific in what you set out to do (the aim), that you detail how you will achieve that aim (the method), that you note any anticipated resources that you will use (support), and that you set a realistic timeframe for completion of the work planned. If someone else will verify your learning, perhaps your personal tutor, make space for their signature in the paperwork. Resist the temptation to set out with grand plans, multiple aims and unrealistic timeframes. Identify fewer achievable aims and progress from there.

Table 11.1: Possible simple portfolio layout

Of the four students whose learning we have reported in this book, Fatima was the most enthusiastic and well organised with regard to her portfolio of learning. We discussed with her the different ways in which her portfolio represented her critical thinking to others. Four things stood out.

- The number of connections made between entries within her portfolio. There were very clear connections made between plans and subsequent evidence of learning, and the cross referencing enabled the reader to follow this path. For example, section 2 entries cross-referenced the relevant section 3 plan and alerted the reader to any additional evidence of achievement within section 1.

- The discrimination shown as regards the number of entries made. Fatima's was not the biggest or heaviest portfolio submitted for assessment but it was the best. She explained:

I knew from the start that I couldn't record every experience and reflection, it would be exhausting. As my portfolio grew the record would become ever more complex! For that reason I started jotting down rough notes on experiences and then writing up only those that stood the test of time, or else combining reflections on several incidents to demonstrate how I brought ideas together.

The portfolio is a working document, so some elements will remain work in rough, while others will become refined – they become part of the end product submitted for assessment.

- The focus of the entries made. These attended closely not only to the learning outcomes set within her course but also to the different sorts of experience she was having. The examiners noted how differently she thought when supporting different groups of patients and working in different settings. She was clearly able to adapt her thinking to context and need.

- The way in which her plans evolved. There was clear evidence of Fatima's quest for knowledge, in her independent study as well as in what others taught or shared. Fatima noted:

I was quite tempted to dump some of my early plans from the portfolio, because they seemed naive. My tutor, though, helped me to see them as an audit trail and helped me to write a short essay that I added at the end, which I called 'journeying'. I got the student prize for insights associated with that work – the way I dealt with uncertainty within my studies.

Activity 11.2	*Critical thinking*

Prepare a single paragraph of writing that you think demonstrates critical thinking, which attends to a stated learning outcome and shows that you are approaching care with due concern for the context or clientele of your practice. To help others to evaluate your paragraph, state the learning outcome above your short piece of work. We have included an excerpt from one of Fatima's portfolio entries at the end of this chapter for you to compare with your own. What do your work and hers have in common? If one entry seems better than the other, why is this?

Next, repeat the process, preparing a short plan for future learning, either one drawn from your own portfolio or one that seems important to you now and you draft from scratch. Refer to Table 11.1 as an aide memoire of what should feature in your plan. What lessons do you draw from a review of your own and Fatima's offering?

Reflection and your portfolio

We discussed the process of reflective writing at some length in Chapter 10, so here we will share more specific thoughts on reflective writing that draw together the individual reflections that you have developed earlier. We call this process 'synthesis of learning' and it can, at best, demonstrate your ability to theorise about nursing care. A simple analogy can help us to demonstrate the value of this. Imagine you are staring up into the night sky and you spot a particularly bright star. You study this star using some binoculars. You learn something about the star, its colour and magnitude of light perhaps. But to make better sense of stars and our position in relation to stars and galaxies, we need to gather together a collection of such observations. We need to spot the position of stars in the sky and to note that stars seem to be clustered more densely in one part of the sky than another. In this way, we learn something about galaxies and, with some extra reading, discover something about our own galaxy and our position within it. The area of dense stars is where we look into the Milky Way and understand our position towards the edge of that galaxy. Linking reflections together can be like the comparison of stars and the realisation that they seem to form some sort of pattern. If we start to recognise patterns, perhaps some that recur again and again, we start to theorise what is happening. We begin to anticipate what we might see next and to speculate about why this happens. Much of what you have already read in this textbook about narratives and discourses in practice relates exactly to this, the search for patterns and what these might mean. You examine your own professional narratives, what you are trying to do and relate them to the narratives that you find around you. You search for discourses, for example those relating to what constitutes more person-centred care.

For such an overarching reflection to work it needs to involve a series of steps.

- Identifying all the relevant experiences and indicating why these constitute a group (Fatima started these entries by listing all the preceding references that were being discussed and stating in a line or two what they were all about. In one instance, this was 'effective listening').

- Comparing and contrasting experiences. This means showing experiences that seem to signal the same thing and others that remind us that neat explanations might not be possible. With regard to effective listening, for instance, Fatima noted that experiences repeatedly emphasised the importance of adequate time, privacy and attention, if listening was to be effective. She noted, however, that patients varied in their need for feedback on what had been understood by the nurse. Some needed the nurse to summarise what had been understood, while others were content that the nurse had simply given of her time.

- Speculating what this tells us. As with individual reflections, we need to determine what (if anything) the experiences tell us. It is necessary at this level, where several reflections are brought together, to be especially cautious about overstating what the experience means. We need to identify the limits of what experience seems to explain, and to note where any resultant, working theory starts to falter. Fatima determined that, while we might ideally wish to provide patients with a summary of what is gleaned from their account of problems or needs, it seemed sometimes sufficient to report back just the highlights. This would be enough to reassure a large number of patients of our appreciation of their needs. There were, however, exceptions to this principle, especially where patients were talking about matters relating to informed consent. There, and in other areas where patient safety was important, it was critical to indicate exactly all that had been understood.

- Determining what follows next. While actions may be possible with reference to individual reflections (e.g., I will not assume that all patients have enough funds to easily secure a balanced diet), further enquiries and discussions may be the more common outcome for reflections that draw on several experiences. This was important in Fatima's example, because the reputation of nurses, as advocates, as carers and as communicators, rested upon how effective listening was understood and used. In her portfolio entry, therefore, she reported that she took the observations to a clinical update meeting for the ward nurses and that it provoked a thoughtful debate. Registered nurse colleagues complimented her on her analysis and started to reflect on their own experiences afresh.

While we can only guess what you deliberate on and what you then conclude, our experience suggests that even quite modest series of experiences can start to generate reflections that might support a very tentative theory on one aspect of practice. We start to identify a narrative, something that explains what we are doing.

Students we have supported have shared narratives on aspects of patient care, on implementing healthcare policy, on the nature of practice innovation and on multidisciplinary working, to name but a few. The subsequent group discussions have then served to modify or augment the narrative and suggest a new round of observations or enquiries that might enable the nurse to test these ideas further. While this reflective entry appears in section 2 of the portfolio, it has often generated a new entry in section 3. Fatima, too, generated a new action plan in association with her reflections on active listening and began to ask patients what they most valued when nurses fed back on the conversations shared with them. She started to search for the recurring, patient-valued elements of feedback by nurses, so that these could be used more frequently in her own practice.

Sharing group discussions about a working narrative enables you to join together reflection and critical thinking. You have begun to formulate ideas about care as a result of several reflections, and the support, challenge and questions that you encounter in group discussion enable you to deepen your analysis. This is frequently how nursing care is refined and improved. One colleague shares an observation with several others and comparisons are made regarding what has been discovered. Each then explores what remains to be understood, what might enhance care and what could be done to improve the knowledge or skill of the practitioner. While research can certainly fuel practice improvements, critically discussed reflections can too. Your portfolio becomes the record of that process.

Activity 11.3 *Critical thinking*

Consider whether, as a result of several learning experiences, those in clinical settings and beyond, you are starting to formulate working narratives, tentative explanations of how nursing works, and what is important in the delivery of nursing care. At best, these are likely to relate to the support of a given patient group, or perhaps to techniques or processes that are used again and again by nurses (e.g., patient education, discharge planning, referral to social service agencies). The focus of your interest should be relatively discrete, as was Fatima's. Follow the above steps to formulate a tentative working narrative that you can share with study group colleagues and your tutor. Your written entry to the portfolio at this stage will be in rough form. It is open to modification as a result of the conversations that you next share with colleagues. There will be opportunity during the study group conversation for you to defend your points, to consider alternative observations and to connect these discoveries to some of the theory that you may have been taught.

Making the case for your development

While your portfolio may be submitted for assessment purposes at one or more points within your course, there is a sense in which it never quite ends as a product. There is always something more that could be added or something that could be modified in the light of a new enquiry or experience. Using your portfolio, though, taking it beyond personal reflection, is vital. If you never share your reflections and claims with others, there is every possibility that you might delude yourself regarding what is important, effective, professional or needful in nursing. There are a number of junctures, therefore, where you share the portfolio with others and use it to make the case regarding your professional development; for example:

- sharing end of module or annual work with your personal tutor (this tutor is interested in the different themes of your development and may make recommendations with regard to these);

- showing work to colleagues at the end of a clinical placement (sometimes mentors are asked to review clinical placement reflections from the portfolio with you);

- submitting the work for gateway assessment (portfolio-based learning is frequently used in nursing and you may need to satisfy portfolio requirements to proceed to the next stage or level of your course);

- demonstrating to others that you have successfully completed a probationary period of practice after registration as a nurse, or on moving into a specialist field of work;

- demonstrating to an employer or other authority that your learning is up to date and that you remain fit to practise, at either a standard or a more advanced practice level.

Requirements vary concerning the contents of the portfolio. For annual appraisal purposes, the post-registration review of your work, or for module assessment purposes, other select elements of the portfolio might need to be submitted and discussed. You may, for example, need to submit records of placement learning outcomes successfully met (with mentor signatures) and a series of reflections that capture your discoveries there. In most instances, personal tutors like to see an overview of your development but, for many others, you will submit an excerpt from your portfolio.

It can feel strange, even unsettling, to share elements of your work after what may have seemed very private reflection. Portfolios of learning, however, remain at least semi-public documents, open to review by examiners and, sometimes, those charged with investigating malpractice. Even if you are not under investigation yourself, you may still hold a record that sheds light on incidents involving another practitioner. We suggest, therefore, that you write the portfolio always as though entries could be inspected by others. It is important to date entries and link them to the places where the experiences were shared. Later, where the law or code of conduct requirements dictate, you may be asked to elaborate on your entries.

A well-structured and organised portfolio will make significant points about your professionalism. It demonstrates your critical thought and reflection. But to use the portfolio to best effect, with a current purpose in mind, you must have read it recently and considered how it addresses the requirements of the day. For example, what within the portfolio points to your abilities as required in a job description? What is it about your portfolio that shows your commitment and interest in a particular field of practice into which you hope to move? Taking time to re-read your portfolio and draw key points from it to add to a letter of application, use in an interview or include within a presentation will enhance your chances of success. The same point holds good in 'open book' examinations, where students are allowed to bring notes, including excerpts from their portfolios, into the examination room. What are the most relevant entries here? There will not be time to find and refer to everything in such settings, so identify what is most pertinent to the requirements of the day.

Activity 11.4   *Critical thinking*

Return to Activity 11.1 and consider whether you should add to your list of bullet points describing the advantages of building a portfolio.

- Had you previously considered how the portfolio can demonstrate your style of reasoning and your attitudes and approach to others? This might be advantageous if your attitudes were subsequently questioned.
- Does it serve to show your inquisitiveness and commitment to learning, something that might be reviewed if you struggled with a certain section of your course or if a special award was being considered?
- Does your portfolio become an important resource when you seek a post in a much-favoured clinical area of practice? Could this provide the edge that helps you to secure the post?

Update your bullet point list now and refer to it periodically if your interest in portfolio building and maintenance starts to flag.

Chapter summary

This chapter has considered what a portfolio consists of and how it relates to the critical thinking and reflection that are so much a part of nursing courses and professional practice. We have made the case that, while building and maintaining a portfolio can seem onerous (especially if you are not naturally inclined towards making diary entries), there are distinct advantages, as well as professional responsibilities, associated with portfolio work. The portfolio has a utilitarian purpose – it can be used as evidence of your achievements, abilities and potential. It becomes a vehicle for enhanced thinking and working, as you start to examine how and why care could or should be different. At best, it fuels the process of theorising – something nurses should engage in wherever they are worried about practice. Writing up reflections that synthesise a series of experiences and past reflections made at the time can help you to think more conceptually and 'out of the box' (i.e., more creatively).

At its very best, building and using a portfolio is not something that you arrange secretively. It becomes part of the fabric of collective learning. You get into the habit of comparing

continued ...

notes with colleagues, reflections, excerpts from what you have read and examples of research evidence that you wish to evaluate and perhaps use. The portfolio is, therefore, a vehicle for professional discourse, which enables us to sustain our interest in nursing and the enrichment of nursing care.

All of this starts with prosaic first steps. You need to arrange the portfolio in a clear, accessible and consistent manner. You need to set up sections and entries in such a way that you can cross-reference material; only then does it enable you to show how you combine insights to demonstrate your understanding. You need to select what goes into the portfolio, accept that some first entries may be tentative or rough, and remain open to adjustment or refinement. Arranging the portfolio in looseleaf or computer-based form provides that kind of flexibility. You can add to the portfolio and take away from it, at will.

In the craft guilds of the Middle Ages, one of the first things an apprentice did was to build or design a tool they would use throughout their career. Their first work was to create a model, a template that guided some of their practice as a master craftsperson. Portfolio building does exactly this. You build a tool for your own use that can serve you well for a long time. It is worth the investment.

Activities: Brief outline answers and reflections

Activity 11.2: Critical thinking (page 175)

Extract from Fatima's critical thinking work

Learning outcome: The student will be able to, in association with the patient and other relevant stakeholders, develop a nursing care plan that reflects relevant priorities and needs.

During my placement on Ivy Ward, I engaged in three episodes of care planning, each with a different patient and experienced nurse in attendance. As this is a surgical ward, with a large number of patients staying with us for relatively short periods of time (2–4 days) and, as there are standard protocols for the majority of care delivered, my individualised care planning centred either on what supplemented the standard protocol or on variations to the protocol mandated by the patient's circumstances. Care planning had to demonstrate due regard for the patient as an individual, determine what was realisable during the hospital stay (other care might be recommended post-discharge) and work with the available resources (other patients competed for our attention, so we needed to plan for the needs of the group as well as the needs of the individual). I noted that, while all the registered nurses recommended slightly different approaches to collaboration in care planning, all were referenced against what I describe as 'practice consequences'. One registered nurse said to me, 'Imagine what would happen if you did do this and what might happen if you didn't. You need to weigh up the benefits and the costs of care, especially if you agree a plan that you expect others to contribute to.' I practised with that idea in mind then, and discovered all three patients appreciated my efforts to personalise care as far as possible. They hadn't expected 'tailor-made care', were well aware of the pressures on hospital beds, but applauded my extra questions: about what the patients did normally, what they found easiest or most worthwhile and what frightened or encouraged them.

Our notes

This ably shows Fatima addressing the learning outcome, as she demonstrates a due regard for patients and acknowledges their part in care planning. In addition, though, there is a clear recognition here of the constraints upon joint care planning. Resources are finite and the plans cannot be unlimited. The stakeholders acknowledged here, then, are the patient, other patients on the ward and the healthcare professionals who must balance the priorities of care. A further benefit of this passage is that she indicates how the learning is achieved – through discussion and observation with three different nurses. This shows how Fatima is able to synthesise information from different sources.

Here is the example of an outline plan Fatima prepared for another element of her learning. Fatima was interested in identifying how nurses on Ivy Ward evaluated their daily care-giving efforts. She believed that feeling good about the shift completed was important if a career was to be sustained in nursing. Several of the nurses seemed hard-pressed in their work but also content with what they achieved.

Aim

To identify what, within care giving in a ward shift, sustains registered nurses in their commitment to nursing work, that is, what gives them personal satisfaction.

Method

1. Observations of selected nurses who share the same shifts as me.
2. Brief discussions with each of them, about what sustains them and helps them to always try to improve their contribution.

Support

The nurses themselves are my chief resource, but I will also look in the library for a textbook on the psychology of work. While that book might not be on nursing, I think it might have something to offer anyway.

Time-frame

I will continue with this work for the remainder of my clinical placement, which is just over a month away.

Achievement proof

I will be able to list three or four key things that help sustain a nurse in their work. To each item on that list I will then add a reflection on the extent to which I have developed same.

Our notes

We were impressed with the clarity and the precision of this plan. It is opportunistic – learning will happen as and when Fatima can observe and speak with the nurses concerned, but the approach is coherent and impressively supported by the idea of dipping into a book on the psychology of work. While it is an unconventional action plan, focusing on the meaning of nursing work rather than clinical skills, we thought it very valid. What sustains a career is interest in what we achieve on a daily basis. We admired the way Fatima has also anticipated what would constitute achievement in this work, which is important given that this is not something routinely assessed by the college.

Further reading

Bolton, G (2014) *Reflective Practice: Writing and professional development*, 4th ed. London: Sage.

Although we recommended this book earlier, we have no qualms about mentioning it again. Chapter 4 (on narrative) is valuable as your portfolio represents a continuing narrative on your learning deliberations. Chapter 5 reminds you that you demonstrate a perspective when you write reflectively (yours will need to address set learning outcomes). Chapter 9 attends to reflective practice journals – the principles described here hold good in nursing too.

Reed, S (2015) *Successful Professional Portfolios for Nursing Students*, 2nd ed. London: Sage/Learning Matters.

Sue Reed provides a readily accessible guide to professional portfolios and their use during and after nurse training. There is a valuable glossary of key terms and guidance on collecting as well as representing evidence of student learning.

Useful websites

https://clippings.me/writing-portfolio-how-to

Writing Portfolios: A How-To Guide

This short guide by Nicholas Holmes is aimed at journalists or creative writers but there is interesting emphasis on design and electronic working. When portfolios were first introduced in nursing, their format was much more prescriptive. Recently, design has become more important in nursing too, so you should find some inspiration here.

www.youtube.com/watch?v=ff7E3ZwNrQA

Self-Reflective Journal Writing.mp4 by Optimal Health Counselling Videos

We have emphasised the utilitarian aspects of building and maintaining a reflective journal but this video emphasises health and wellbeing benefits too. The case is made that expressive writing not only demonstrates learning achievements but also materially alters how we think. It is worth noting that journals are used to therapeutic purpose too.

References

Ailey, S, Lamb, K, Friese, T and Christopher, B (2015) Educating nursing students in clinical leadership. *Nursing Management (UK)*, 21(9): 23–8.

Allen, D (2015) *The Invisible Work of Nurses: Hospitals, organisation and healthcare.* Abingdon: Routledge.

Anderson, LW, Krathwohl, DR, Airaisian, PW, Cruickshank, KA, Mayer, RE, Pintrich, PR, Raths, J and Wittrock, MC (2001) *A Taxonomy for Learning, Teaching and Assessing: A revision of Bloom's taxonomy of educational objectives.* Boston, MA: Pearson.

Ashby, C (2006) Models for reflective practice. *Practice Nurse*, 32(10): 28–32.

Atherton, I and Kyle, R (2015) Stepping outside your comfort zone. *Nursing Standard*, 29(21): 24–5.

Balasubramanian, B, Chase, S, Nutting, P, Cohen, D, Strickland, P, Crosson, J, William, L and Crabtree, B (2010) Using learning teams for reflective adaptation (ULTRA): insights from a team-based change management strategy in primary care. *Annals of Family Medicine*, 8(5): 425–32.

Baxter Magolda, M (1992) *Knowing and Reasoning in College Students: Gender-related patterns in students' intellectual development.* San Francisco, CA: Jossey-Bass.

Baylis, D (2015) How to avoid negligence claims. *Practice Nurse*, 45(1): 10–11

Benner, P (2001) *From Novice to Expert: Excellence and power in clinical nursing practice.* Commemorative ed. Upper Saddle River, NJ: Prentice Hall.

Bennett, M and McGowan, B (2014) Assessment matters: mentors need support in their role. *British Journal of Nursing*, 23(9): 454–8.

Bergevin, R (2014) Assessing wounds in palliative care. *Nursing*, 44(8): 68–9.

Berry, G (2011) Lesson 3: Sorting main ideas and details with the 'T' method. Available at: https://www.youtube.com/watch?v=WBrR4UHq2Ck

Bloom, B, Engelhart, M, Furst, E, Hill, W and Krathwohl, D (1956) *Taxonomy of Educational Objectives: The classification of educational goals. Handbook 1: Cognitive Domain.* New York: David McKay.

Brown, T, Thornton, T and Stewart, M (2012) *Challenges and Solutions: Narratives of patient centred care.* London: Radcliffe.

Buckwell-Nutt, K, Francis-Shama, J and Kellett, P (2014) A framework for pre-qualifying nurses to build leadership skills. *Nursing Management (UK)*, 21(7): 16–22.

Bulman, C and Schutz, S (2008) *Reflective Practice in Nursing*, 4th ed. Oxford: Blackwell.

Bunniss, S and Kelly, D (2010) Research paradigms in medical education. *Medical Education*, 44: 358–66.

Carr, V, Sangiorgi, D, Buscher, M, Junginger, S and Cooper, R (2011) Integrating evidence-based design and experience based approaches in health service design. *HERD*, 4(4): 12–33.

Carter, A, Sidebotham, M, Creedy, D, Debra, K, Fenwick, J and Gamble, J (2014) Using root-cause analysis to promote critical thinking in final year Bachelor of Midwifery students. *Nurse Education Today*, 34(6): 1018–23.

Christensen, M (2011) Advancing nursing practice: redefining the theoretical and practical integration of knowledge. *Journal of Clinical Nursing*, 20: 873–81.

Clarke, T, Kelleher, M and Fairbrother, G (2010) Starting a care improvement journey: focusing on the essentials of bedside nursing care in an Australian teaching hospital. *Journal of Clinical Nursing*, 19(13/14): 1812–20.

Cohen, S (2013) Talk it and walk it: staff communication, *Nursing Management (USA)*, 44(6): 16–18.

Connor, M and Norman, P (2005) *Predicting Health Behaviour*. Maidenhead: Open University Press/McGraw Hill.

Cortazzi, M and Jin, L (1997) Communicating for learning across cultures, in McNamara, D and Harris, R (eds) *Overseas Students in Higher Education: Issues in teaching and learning*. Abingdon: Routledge, pp. 76–90.

Craig, C (2009) Learning about reflections through exploring narrative enquiry. *Reflective Practice*, 10(1): 105–16.

de Bono, E (2009) *Six Thinking Hats: Run better meetings, make faster decisions*. London: Penguin.

Department of Health and NHS Commissioning Board (2012) *Compassion in Practice: Nursing, midwifery and care staff, our vision and strategy*. London: NHS Commissioning Board.

Dolan, G, Strodl, E and Hamernik, E (2012) Why renal nurses cope so well with their workplace stressors. *Journal of Renal Care*, 38(4): 222–32.

Dovi, G (2015) Empowering change with traditional and virtual journal clubs. *Nursing Management (USA)*, 46(1): 46–50.

Earle, V (2010) Phenomenology as research method or substantive metaphysics? An overview of phenomenology's uses in nursing. *Nursing Philosophy*, 11(4): 286–96.

Ellis, P (ed.) (2013a) *Evidence-Based Practice in Nursing*, 2nd ed. London: Sage/Learning Matters.

Ellis, P (2013b) *Understanding Research for Nursing Students*, 2nd ed. London: Sage/Learning Matters.

Eriksen, K, Dahl, H, Karlsson, B and Arman, M (2014) Strengthening practical wisdom: mental health workers' learning and development. *Nursing Ethics*, 21(6): 707–19.

Fink, D (2009) A self-directed guide to designing courses for significant learning. Norman, OK: Dee Fink and Associates. Available at: www.deefinkandassociates.com/index.php/resources

Francis, R (2013) *Report of the Mid Staffordshire NHS Foundation Trust Public Inquiry, chaired by Robert Francis QC. Presented to Parliament pursuant to Section 26 of the Inquiries Act 2005. HC 898. 3 vols.* London: Stationery Office. Available at: http://webarchive.nationalarchives.gov.uk/20150407084003/http://www.midstaffs-publicinquiry.com/report

Freeborn, D and Knafl, K (2014) Growing up with cerebral palsy: perceptions of the influence of family. *Child, Care, Health and Development*, 40(5): 671–9.

Furberg, B and Furberg, C (2007) *Evaluating Clinical Research: All that glitters is not gold*, 2nd ed. New York: Springer.

Gabby, J and Le May, A (2011) *Practice-Based Evidence for Healthcare: Clinical mindlines*. Abingdon: Routledge.

Game, E (2014) Blowing the whistle: what are your rights? *British Journal of Neuroscience Nursing*, 10(1): 46–7.

Gibbs, G (1988) *Learning By Doing: A guide to teaching and learning methods.* Oxford: Oxford Polytechnic Further Education Unit.

Gobet, F (2005) Chunking models of expertise: implications for education. *Applied Cognitive Psychology*, 19: 183–204.

Gobet, F and Chassey, P (2008) Towards an alternative to Benner's theory of expert intuition in nursing: a discussion paper. *International Journal of Nursing Studies*, 45(1): 129–39.

Green, J and Thorogood, N (2004) *Qualitative Methods for Health Research.* London: Sage.

Guardiola-Wanden-Berghe, R, Gil-Perez, J, Sanz-Valero, J and Wanden-Berghe, C (2011) Evaluating the quality of websites relating to diet and eating disorders. *Health Information and Libraries Journal*, 28(4): 294–301.

Haigh, C and Costa, C (2013) Information about assisted dying: an evaluation of web-based information resources. *Journal of Research in Nursing*, 18(5): 471–80.

Hamilton, G, Ortega, R, Hochstetler, V, Pierson, K, Lin, P and Lowes, S (2014) Teaching communication skills to hospice teams: comparing the effectiveness of a communications skill laboratory with In-Person, Second Life, and phone role-playing. *Journal of Hospice and Palliative Medicine*, 31(6): 611–18.

Hammond, K (1978) Towards increasing competence of thought in public policy formation, in Hammond, K (ed.) *Judgement and Decision in Public Policy Formation.* Boulder, CO: Westview Press, pp. 11–32.

Hammond, K (1996) *Human Judgement and Social Policy: Irreducible uncertainty, inevitable error, unavoidable justice.* Oxford: Oxford University Press.

Hammond, K (2007) *Beyond Rationality: The sources for wisdom in a troubled time.* New York: Oxford University Press.

Hasson, F, McKenna, H and Keeney, S (2013) Delegating and supervising unregistered professionals: the student nurse experience. *Nurse Education Today*, 33(3): 229–35.

Honey, M and Doherty, I (2014) Research brief: using a wiki to support student nurses learning discipline specific health terminology. *Nursing Praxis in New Zealand*, 30(1): 42–3.

Honey, P and Mumford, A (1982) *Manual of Learning Styles.* London: PeterHoney.com.

Howatson-Jones, L (2016) *Reflective Practice in Nursing*, 3rd ed. London: Sage/Learning Matters.

Hsu, M and McCormack, B (2012) Using narrative inquiry with older people to inform practice and service developments. *Journal of Clinical Nursing*, 21(5/6): 841–9.

Hudson, B (2015) Can GPs coordinate 'whole person care'? *Journal of Integrated Care*, 23(1): 10–16.

Hudson, K (2014) Teaching nursing concepts through an online discussion board. *Journal of Nursing Education*, 53(9): 531–6.

Joel, L (2009) *Advanced Practice in Nursing: Essentials for role development*, 2nd ed. Philadelphia, PA: FA Davis.

Johns, C (1995) Framing learning through reflection within Carper's fundamental ways of knowing in nursing. *Journal of Advanced Nursing*, 22: 226–34.

Karlsson, E, Savenstedt, S, Axelsson, K and Zingmark, K (2014) Stories about life narrated by people with Alzheimer's disease. *Journal of Advanced Nursing*, 70(12): 2791–9.

Kelton, M (2014) Clinical coaching: an innovative role to improve marginal nursing students' clinical practice. *Nurse Education in Practice*, 14: 709–13.

Kilbride, C, Perry, L, Flatley, M, Turner, E and Meyer, J (2011) Developing theory and practice: creation of a community of practice through action research produced excellence in stroke care. *Journal of Interprofessional Care*, 25(2): 91–4.

Koharchik, L, Caputi, L, Robb, M, and Culleitin, A (2015) Fostering clinical reasoning in nursing students. *American Journal of Nursing*, 115(1): 58–61.

Kothari, A, Rudman, D, Dobbins, M, Rouse, M, Sibbald, S and Edwards, N (2012) The use of tacit and explicit knowledge in public health: a qualitative study. *Implementation Science*, 7(1): 20–31.

Kuhn, T (2012) *The Structure of Scientific Revolutions*, 50th anniversary ed. Chicago, IL: University of Chicago Press.

Lancaster, J, Wong, A and Roberts, S (2012) Tech versus talk: a comparison study of two different lecture styles within a Master of Science nurse practitioner course. *Nurse Education Today*, 32(5): e14–18.

Larchman, V (2012) Applying the ethics of care to your nursing practice. *Medical-Surgical Nursing*, 21(2): 112–16.

Little, C (2012) Patient expectations of 'effectiveness' in healthcare: an example from medical herbalism. *Journal of Clinical Nursing*, 21(5/6): 718–27.

Long, M, Bekelman, D and Make, B (2014) Improving quality of life in chronic obstructive pulmonary disease by integrating approaches to dyspnoea, anxiety and depression. *Journal of Hospice and Palliative Nursing*, 16(8): 514–20.

Lorette, K (2012) *The Complete Guide to Running Successful Workshops and Seminars: Everything you need to know to plan, promote and present a conference explained.* Ocala, FL: Atlantic.

Lovatt, A (2014) Defining critical thoughts. *Nurse Education Today*, 34(5): 670–2.

Lowth, M (2014) The child with abdominal pain. *Practice Nurse*, 44(9): 10–13.

Lucas, R (2009) *Training Workshop Essentials: Designing, developing and delivering learning events that get results.* San Francisco, CA: Pfeiffer.

Maio, G and Haddock, G (2009) *The Psychology of Attitudes and Attitude Change*, 2nd ed. London: Sage.

Manookian, A, Cheraghi, M and Nasrabadi, A (2014) Factors influencing patients' dignity: a qualitative study. *Nursing Ethics*, 21(3): 323–34.

Martensson, G and Lofmark, A (2013) Implementation and student evaluation of clinical final examination in nursing education. *Nurse Education Today*, 33(12): 1563–8.

Martin, G (2015) Obesity in question: understandings of body shape, self and normalcy among children in Malta. *Sociology of Health and Illness*, 37(2): 212–26.

Mason, V, Leslie, G, Clark, K, Lyons, P, Walke, E, Butler, C and Griffin, M (2014) Compassion fatigue, moral distress and work engagement in surgical intensive care unit trauma nurses: a pilot study. *Dimensions of Critical Care Nursing*, 33(4): 215–25.

McCarthy, B, Andrews, T and Hegarty, J (2015) Emotional resistance building: how family members of loved ones undergoing chemotherapy treatment process their fear of emotional collapse. *Journal of Advanced Nursing*, 71(4): 837–48.

McNett, S (2012) Teaching nursing psychomotor skills in a fundamentals laboratory: a literature review. *Nursing Education Perspectives*, 33(5): 328–33.

Moon, J (2008) *Critical Thinking: An exploration of theory and practice.* Abingdon: Routledge.

Morley, D (2012) Enhancing networking and proactive learning skills in the first year university experience through the use of wikis. *Nurse Education Today*, 32(3): 261–6.

Morrall, P and Goodman, B (2013) Critical thinking, nurse education and universities: some thoughts on current issues and implications for nursing practice. *Nurse Education Today*, 33(9): 935–7.

Moule, P and Goodman, M (2014) *Nursing Research: An introduction*, 2nd ed. London: Sage.

Mulnix, J (2012) Thinking critically about critical thinking. *Educational Philosophy and Theory*, 44(5): 464–79.

Norris, M and Gimber, P (2013) Developing nursing students' metacognitive skills using social technology. *Teaching and Learning in Nursing*, 8(1): 17–21.

Nursing and Midwifery Council (2010) *Standards for Pre-registration Nursing Education.* London: NMC.

Nursing and Midwifery Council (2015) *The Code: Professional standards of practice and behaviour for nurses and midwives.* London: NMC.

Odell, M (2015) Detection and management of the deteriorating ward patient: an evaluation of nursing practice. *Journal of Clinical Nursing*, 24(1–2): 173–82.

Olsen, N (2013) Self-reflection: foundation of meaningful nursing practice. *Reflection on Nursing Leadership*, 39(2): 1–4.

Padden, M (2013) A pilot study to determine the validity and reliability of the level of reflection on action assessment. *Journal of Nursing Education*, 52(7): 410–15.

Paley, J (2014) Heidegger, lived experience and method. *Journal of Advanced Nursing*, 70(7): 1520–31.

Pearson, A, Field, J and Jordan, Z (2007) *Evidence-Based Clinical Practice in Nursing and Healthcare: A comprehensive approach to evidence-based practice in nursing and the health professions.* Oxford: Blackwell.

Pilcher, J (2014) Problem-based learning in the NICU. *Neonatal Network*, 33(4): 221–4.

Pitt, V, Powis, D, Levett-Jones, T and Hunter, S (2015) The influence of critical thinking skills on performance and progression in a pre registration nursing program. *Nurse Education Today*, 35(1): 125–31.

Plested, M (2014) Mindful midwifery: a phenomenological paradigm. *Practising Midwife*, 17(11): 18–20.

Price, B (2003) Academic voices and the challenges of tutoring. *Nurse Education Today*, 23(8): 628–37.

Price, B (2009) Supporting patients' dignity in the community. *Primary Health Care*, 19(3): 40–7.

Price, B (2011a) Making better use of older people's narratives. *Nursing Older People*, 23(6): 31–7.

Price, B (2011b) Improving clinical reasoning in children's nursing through narrative analysis. *Nursing Children and Young People*, 23(6): 28–34.

References

Price, B (2012) Key principles in assessing students' practice-based learning. *Nursing Standard*, 26(49): 49–55.

Price, B (2013) Understanding nursing 'nous' in the context of service improvements. *Nursing Management (UK)*, 20(14): 28–35.

Quality Assurance Agency for Higher Education (2008) *The Framework for Higher Education in England, Wales and Northern Ireland*. Mansfield: QAA. Available at: www.qaa.ac.uk/publications/information-and-guidance/publication?PubID=2718#.VfU8y3hfUQ4

Quality Assurance Agency Scotland (2014) *The Framework for Qualifications of Higher Education Institutes in Scotland*. Glasgow: QAA. Available at: http://www.qaa.ac.uk/publications/information-and-guidance/publication?PubID=2674#.VfU8BnhfUQ5

Quinn, F and Hughes, S (2013) *Quinn's Principles and Practice of Nurse Education*, 6th ed. London: Thomson Learning.

Rankin, B (2013) Emotional intelligence: enhancing value-based practice and compassionate care in nursing. *Journal of Advanced Nursing*, 69(12): 2717–25.

Ransom, E, Joshi, M, Nash, D and Ransom, S (2008) *The Healthcare Quality Handbook: Vision, strategy and tools*, 2nd ed. Washington, DC: Hap Alpha.

Reed, S (2015) *Successful Professional Portfolios for Nursing Students*, 2nd ed. London: Sage/Learning Matters.

Roberts, L (2010) Health information and the internet: the 5 Cs website evaluation tool. *British Journal of Nursing*, 19(5): 322–5.

Rolfe, G (2006) Judgements without rules: towards a postmodern ironist concept of research validity. *Nursing Enquiry*, 13(1): 7–15.

Rolfe, G and Jasper, M (2010) *Critical Reflection in Practice: Generating Knowledge for Care*. Basingstoke: Palgrave Macmillan.

Schlegel, C, Woermann, U, Shaha, M, Rethan, S and Van der Vleutin, C (2012) Effects of communication training on real practice performance: a role play module versus a standardized patient module. *Journal of Nursing Education*, 51(1): 16–22.

Schön, D (1987) *Educating the Reflective Practitioner*. San Francisco, CA: Jossey-Bass.

Scott, K and McSherry, R (2009) Evidence-based nursing: clarifying the concepts for nurses in practice. *Journal of Clinical Nursing*, 18(8): 1085–95.

Sharples, K (2011) *Successful Practice Learning for Nursing Students*, 2nd ed. Exeter: Learning Matters.

Spiers, J, Williams, B, Gibson, B, Kabatoff, W, McIlwraith, D, Sculley, A and Richard, E (2014) Graduate nurses' learning trajectories and experiences of problem-based learning: a focused ethnography study. *International Journal of Nursing Studies*, 51(11): 1462–71.

Standing, M (2014) *Clinical Judgement and Decision Making for Nursing Students*, 2nd ed. London: Sage/Learning Matters.

Swatridge, C (2014) *Oxford Guide to Effective Argument and Critical Thinking*. Oxford: Oxford University Press.

Van den Brink-Budgen, R (2010) *Critical Thinking for Students: Learn the skills of analysing, evaluating and producing arguments*, 4th ed. Begbroke: How to Books.

Weaver, K and Olson, J (2006) Understanding paradigms used for nursing research. *Journal of Advanced Nursing*, 53(4): 459–69.

Wyer, P, Silva, S, Post, S and Quinlan, P (2014) Relationship-centred care: antidote, guide post or blind alley? The epistemology of 21st century health care. *Journal of Evaluation in Clinical Practice*, 20(6): 881–9.

Zehler, J (2015) The 5 gallon bucket. *Journal of Emergency Nursing*, 41(1): 71–3.

Index